CW01638195

Raising Light

A Memoir of Faith, Family, and the Miracles That Shape Us

Lindsey Vesnic

© 2026 Lindsey Erin Vesnic

All rights reserved. No part of this publication may be reproduced, stored in a retrieval system, or transmitted in any form or by any means —electronic, mechanical, photocopying, recording, or otherwise— without the prior written permission of the author.

Photography

Interior and cover photography by Cindy Valentine Photography

Used with permission. All rights reserved.

Published by

Meridian Book Publishers

605 Third Avenue, 43rd Floor

New York, NY 10158

info@meridianbookpublishers.com

Senior Project & Marketing Manager: Ronald Grayson

Senior Writer/Editor: Michelle Mourton

ISBNs

Paperback: 979-8295466281

Hardcover: 979-8295466519

Printed in Chambersburg, PA and/or LaVergne, TN, USA

For more information visit: https://raisinglightmama.com/

Contents

Part 4: Choosing Light in a Complicated World

Part 5: Full Circle

To my children,

Lucy and Anderson—you are the brightest lights I've ever known. This book exists because of you.

To Richard,

my greatest gift on this side of Heaven—your love, humor, and loyalty anchor me every day. Thank you for believing in me before I believed in myself.

To Amy Masko,

who saw the light in me when I was still stumbling through shadows. You didn't just change my academic path—you changed my life. Thank you for reminding me that dyslexia didn't disqualify me from this calling; it prepared me for it.

And **to every parent, teacher, and child** who's ever been told they're too much or not enough—this is for you.

A Note from the Author

This book is not a manual.

It's a mosaic.

A collection of moments—messy, miraculous, and deeply meaningful—that led me to discover that the most sacred kind of learning begins at home. Not because home is perfect. But because home is personal.

You'll read a lot about Lucy in these pages. That's not because I love her more. It's simply a matter of time. I've had the honor of being with her every day since she was born—nursing her, watching her take her first steps, and learning to read side by side on our living room floor.

But this story isn't only hers.

It's also about Anderson—my stepson, who taught me what it means to love with no strings attached. You'll meet him throughout the book, and though his chapters may look different, his light is just as bright.

It's also about Richard, my husband and partner in all things. And it's about me—the woman I was before motherhood, and the one I've become since. It's about growing up with dyslexia, falling in love unexpectedly, and finding God's fingerprints in the folds of everyday life.

This book is about learning. Not just the kind that happens in workbooks or lesson plans—but the kind that shapes who we are. The kind that happens when a parent shows up, pays attention, and chooses to nurture—not rush—a child's unfolding mind.

And if this book finds you somewhere in the middle of your own story—tired, uncertain, or simply trying to raise your kids with a little more light—

Then know this:

You're not alone.

And I'm so glad you're here.

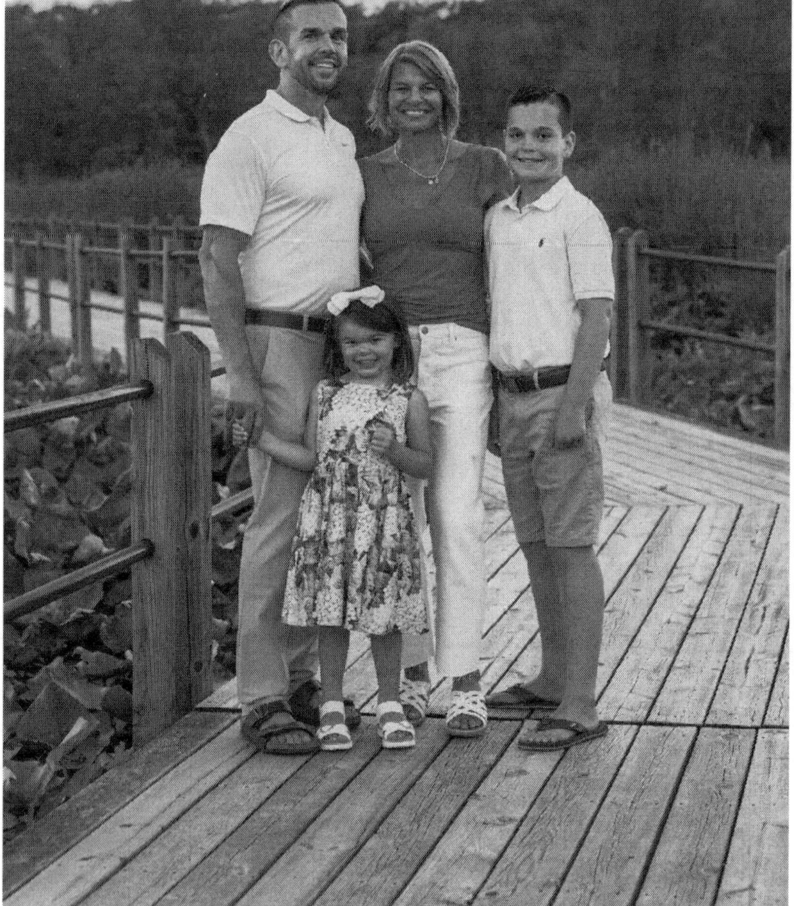

Prologue

"The light shines in the darkness, and the darkness has not overcome it."

—John 1:5

I've always loved the word light.

It's in the laughter of my children, the glow of the late afternoon sun, the warmth of a room filled with music and memory. Light draws us in, lifts our spirits, and helps us see what's truly there. It reveals. It comforts. It shows the way forward.

So when I sat down to write this book, I kept coming back to that word.

I'm not raising perfect children.

I'm raising light.

Light doesn't compete—it shines.

Light doesn't rush—it radiates.

Light doesn't need to prove anything—it simply illuminates.

This book isn't about how to raise a gifted child or how to replicate someone else's journey. It's about the sacred work of helping a child become who they were made to be. It's about education, yes—but more than that, it's about presence. About noticing the spark. About protecting wonder. About choosing consistency over comparison, and curiosity over control.

In our home, learning isn't something we squeeze in. It's the air we breathe.

We read. We wrestle. We talk about God and grace and why caterpillars turn into butterflies. We make mistakes and try again. We go outside and notice things—tiny things, wild things, beautiful things. We find joy in the ordinary, and when something isn't working, we don't force it. We slow down and listen.

Because light doesn't grow under pressure.

It grows when it's nurtured.

So this is our story. A story about learning and love, parenting and purpose. A story about one family's journey toward raising children with intention, depth, and joy. It's not always tidy or easy—but it's always honest. And it's full of light.

Part 1: Foundations of Faith, Family, and Becoming

Before we can raise light in someone else, we have to find it within ourselves.

This first part is my story. It's not the one I planned to tell. If I'm honest, I didn't want to start here—but I know I have to. Because becoming a parent doesn't begin in the hospital or at a baby shower, it begins in the quiet, often painful places where we were once small. Where we were shaped. Where we had to fight to be seen and heard. Where we learned what love is—and what it isn't.

My journey to motherhood started with healing.

It started with learning to see myself not through the world's eyes, but through God's. It started with naming my wounds, reclaiming my worth, and slowly, intentionally, becoming the kind of person I needed when I was young.

Before I could raise a child, I had to be raised again myself.

Chapter 1

From the Ugly Duckling

"But God chose the foolish things of the world to shame the wise… the weak things of the world to shame the strong."

—1 Corinthians 1:27

I was born with dyslexia. But I didn't know that right away, of course.

What I did know—what I felt in the very core of my being—was that learning was hard. Reading, writing, math, even directions on a worksheet that seemed so simple to everyone else… they tangled up in my head like spaghetti. By second grade, it was painfully clear to my teachers, my parents, and certainly to me: something was different.

That's when the testing happened. The diagnosis came back. Dyslexia.

Back then, the educational landscape didn't offer much empathy, let alone tailored support, for kids who learned differently. I wasn't handed a learning plan or a team of compassionate teachers. I was handed labels. And whether spoken aloud or not, the message I absorbed was this: "You're going to have to work harder than everyone else just to keep up. And you still might not."

Letters and numbers would flip around right before my eyes. My brain seemed to toss them like puzzle pieces, never quite putting them back in the right order. You can imagine how that makes reading a challenge. But worse yet—how crushing it feels when you follow every step in a math problem, only to reverse a digit and get the answer wrong. Over and over. Even when you're trying your hardest.

It's the kind of discouragement that burrows deep into a child's heart. I wasn't lazy. I wasn't incapable. But I was growing up in a system that didn't know how to speak my language. I graduated high school with a mix of C's and D's, feeling tired and small. Invisible.

I also became incredibly shy and unsure of myself. I often stayed quiet even when I had something to say. I didn't trust my thoughts or my words, and I rarely volunteered in class. I wasn't trying to stand out—I was just trying to survive.

Still, I wasn't ready to give up. I wanted more—not just for me, but for kids like me. So I enrolled in a community college, determined to earn enough credits to transfer to a university. My grades weren't perfect, but I finally made it. Two years later, I transferred to a university where everything changed.

Her name was Amy Masko.

She was my professor in the English department. (Yes—English. I was an English Education major, which still astonishes people when they learn I was dyslexic.) Amy taught ENG 400, a senior-level course called Critical Issues in the Language Arts. And dyslexia? That was certainly a critical issue.

When our big assignment was announced—a semester-long action research paper—I felt defeated before I even began. The original topic was differentiated instruction, and I didn't even know where to start. I approached her after class, trying to explain that I was overwhelmed, that I had dyslexia, that I wasn't sure I could manage this paper.

She gave me a long, quiet look. Not a pitying one. Not annoyed. It was as if she was peering through every excuse and straight into my potential.

Then she asked, "Do you know what dyslexia is?"

I blinked, taken aback. Of course, I knew. I lived it.

But she listened to my explanation, then gently interrupted and said, "You now have a one-week extension. But only because you have new work to do. You're going to research dyslexia. It's due next week."

I left irritated and confused… but also curious. And so, I dug in. What I found stunned me.

Einstein. Picasso. Leonardo da Vinci. Agatha Christie. Walt Disney. Steven Spielberg.

All dyslexic.

It felt like my soul had been jolted awake. For the first time, I saw my diagnosis not as a limitation—but as a lens. A signature.

Something I shared with some of the greatest minds and creators in history.

The next day, I turned in my research. Professor Masko looked at me and asked, "What did you discover?"

A bit sheepishly, I told her: "A lot of brilliant people were dyslexic."

She smiled. "They weren't just brilliant. They were geniuses. Lindsey, you are a genius."

That moment changed me.

It cracked something open inside. And immediately, I thought of The Ugly Duckling. A little bird who never quite fit in—until he realized he was never meant to. He was something else entirely. Something beautiful.

I completed that paper on differentiated instruction—successfully. What I didn't know was that Amy had submitted it to a national literacy seminar. Thousands applied. Only five students were selected to present.

And somehow, mine was chosen.

The dyslexic girl who had once been told she'd never amount to much was now standing in front of an auditorium full of educators… teaching them.

From that moment on, I soared. Confidence in one area spilled into every other. Even math started to make sense to me—when I stopped believing I was inherently bad at it. I made the Dean's List every semester. I graduated magna cum laude. I was invited to join the Sigma Tau Delta English Honor Society.

Me. A dyslexic English honors student.

It still gives me goosebumps.

But what gives me even more joy is that this journey didn't stop with me. It set the stage for how I would raise my son and my daughter—and how I would build a world of learning that didn't just tolerate difference, but celebrated it.

Because now I knew: I wasn't alone. And I was never broken.

Reflections Pages

1. A moment from this chapter that stood out to me:

____

____

____

2. How this moment connects to my own story, family, or childhood:

____

____

____

3. A belief, habit, or pattern I noticed in myself:

____

____

____

4. A more compassionate or truthful way of seeing this part of my story is:

____

____

____

____

5. One practical step I want to take this week is:

____

____

____

6. What might get in the way:

____

____

____

7. How I can support myself when it feels hard:

____

____

____

8. A Bible verse this chapter reminds me of and why:

____

____

____

9. A prayer, affirmation, or intention I want to carry forward:

____

____

____

Take what serves you, release what doesn't. Healing and learning are slow, holy work — and you are doing beautifully.

Chapter 2

Becoming Me

"And we know that in all things God works for the good of those who love him."

—Romans 8:28

When I crossed the stage at my university graduation—magna cum laude with honors—I felt like I had climbed a mountain no one thought I could scale. I had become a woman I barely recognized—a woman who could speak in front of hundreds, whose name was printed in programs, who was called "gifted." But even in that moment of triumph, I didn't feel like I had arrived. I felt like I had begun.

What followed were years of unexpected detours and deeply formative chapters—each one seeming, at first, like a separate story. But later I'd come to see it all differently. None of it was random. God had a plan. Every career, every calling, was quietly sculpting me into the kind of mother—and teacher—I would one day need to be.

***

Wildlife Rehabilitator

While still in college, my first meaningful job wasn't really a job at all—it was more like volunteer work. And it wasn't in a classroom. It was in the woods, in barns, and in back rooms filled with incubators and the rhythmic hum of heat lamps. I became a wildlife rehabilitator.

It didn't happen by choice, exactly—it felt more like divine intervention. One day, our family dog discovered a baby squirrel, so tiny she didn't even have fur yet. Her eyes were still closed, and she was crawling with fleas. I couldn't walk away. My heart simply wouldn't let me. With no experience and only instinct to guide me, I dove into research, trying everything I could to save her life. I even made a special hammock that wrapped around my neck so I could keep her close at all times. Miraculously, she survived. I named her Chinook.

We shared a beautiful bond, and through her, I learned more than I ever could've imagined. Because of Chinook, I connected with licensed wildlife rehabilitators in my area and eventually became a subpermittee under one of them. I bottle-fed baby squirrels, rescued orphaned raccoons, and learned how to hydrate animals with subcutaneous injections. I taught raccoons how to fish. I massaged paralyzed limbs to restore nerve function—hour after hour, doing whatever was needed. I learned how to earn the trust of wild animals and how to gently prepare them for release back into their natural world.

It was messy, heartbreaking, heartwarming, sacred work.

What I didn't realize at the time was how deeply it was shaping me—especially my ability to observe. Real observation. Not just noticing what an animal did, but understanding why. I learned how to sit quietly with something frightened, without rushing to fix it. I learned the power of patience, the necessity of gentle boundaries, and the difference between helping and interfering. These weren't lessons I read in a textbook. They were earned by showing up every day, watching, listening, and learning.

And surprisingly, learning to read animal behavior gave me a profound understanding of human behavior, too.

Looking back, it's obvious this moment was planted by God. He wanted me to gain the skills I would need in the years to come—and so He sent Chinook to find me. I still see the echoes of that season in the way I parent today. Especially in the quiet moments, when a child is melting down and what they need isn't punishment or a pep talk—but presence and leadership.

***

Dog Trainer

After wildlife work, I shifted toward a path that eventually became its own small business: dog training. For over a decade, I worked with dogs and coached families on everything from basic obedience to serious behavioral issues.

One of my most memorable cases was a pit bull named Charlie. Charlie was the worst ambassador for his breed—aggressive toward anything that moved. On walks, he'd lunge at people, bikes, you name it. Everyone saw him as the problem. But after just one observation, I saw something different. In the dog world, eye contact can be viewed as a challenge—and when fear is added to the equation, you get trouble. People weren't just seeing a dog. They were seeing a "scary pit bull." And Charlie was becoming what they expected him to be.

I had to teach Charlie how to walk properly, of course. But more than that, I had to help people see him differently. I don't know how I came up with the idea, but I had his owners buy him a clown collar. Silly? Definitely. But when you put a clown collar on anything, it looks ridiculous—in the best way. I needed people to look at Charlie and say, "Oh my goodness, look at that cute dog!" And they did. It worked. The clown collar softened people's assumptions and gave Charlie a new label. A better one.

Maybe I knew what that felt like. I had carried the dyslexia label like a burden, like a shadow everyone told me to hide behind. Charlie was doing the same—until someone changed the story. Once people saw him differently—and once his owners stepped up as calm, confident leaders—Charlie became the dog he was meant to be—a true ambassador, at last.

That transformation stayed with me.

What surprised me most about dog training was how much of it wasn't about dogs. It was about people. Teaching them to read body language, to lead with confidence, and to set clear boundaries. Dog training is a misnomer—it's people training. And it made me a better communicator, a better observer, a better teacher. It taught me how to teach by doing, how to adjust when things didn't go to plan, and how to celebrate tiny wins. I learned the power of clear expectations and gentle authority—two things I didn't yet know I'd need every single day as a mother and homeschooler.

There's something sacred about being assertive—not dominant, not fearful. Just assertive. That became a core philosophy of mine, long before I had a child of my own.

***

Teacher

Eventually, I returned to the classroom—this time as a certified teacher. It was a full-circle moment. I, the girl once failed by school, was now shaping it from the inside.

I poured my heart into it. I differentiated lessons for kids who needed a different pace or perspective. I spotted the signs of dyslexia before a label ever hit the file. I kept fidget tools and doodle pads handy. I saw myself in so many of those kids—and I never let them shrink.

My focus was middle schoolers with learning disabilities. Many were on the autism spectrum or had ADD/ADHD. I butted heads with principals more than once. Dog training had taught me to address everything, and I did. If a student stepped out of line, I responded—every single time. And the moment they corrected, we were good. Dog training taught me that, too. You correct, then move forward. No grudges. No lingering shame.

I also expected a lot from my students—probably more than some administrators thought was appropriate. But in my experience, nothing holds a brilliant mind back more than low expectations. I refused to be the person who told a child what they couldn't do.

Then the test scores came in.

On the NWEA standardized test, the average growth rate for a "typical" student is about 12%. My students—those labeled and underestimated—averaged 44% growth. That's not just good. That's astronomical.

But the longer I taught, the more tension I felt. I saw how often the system left little room for individual brilliance. I started dreaming of something freer, more connected—something deeply responsive to each child's unique needs. I wasn't ready to give up teaching. But I was beginning to imagine what education could look like outside the box.

Realtor

At one point, in what felt like a radical shift, I became a Realtor. People are often surprised by that one. But I loved it. I loved helping families find "home"—especially during tender, transitional times. And frankly, I needed something that paid better than teaching.

Real estate taught me how to guide people through big, emotional decisions. I worked with nervous clients, high-stress timelines, and moments full of both fear and hope. I learned to stay grounded, ask better questions, read between the lines, and trust my gut. I also learned how to run a business, manage my own time, and move through uncertainty with grace.

And maybe most importantly, I learned that "home" isn't a place. It's a feeling. One I wanted to create for my own future child.

The Shift

Through all of these chapters, a quiet yearning was growing in the background—a longing to become a mother. I don't speak about that part lightly. The waiting. The prayers. The unspoken grief of months turning into years.

That story deserves its own space—and it will have one. But what I want to say here is this: when Lucy finally came into our lives, I didn't feel like I had stepped away from my career. I felt like I had stepped into my calling.

I hadn't abandoned everything I'd worked for. I had been preparing for it.

The tenderness and patience of wildlife rehabilitation. The intuition and assertiveness of dog training. The insight of teaching. The structure and confidence of real estate. All of it came with me into motherhood.

And this time, I wouldn't have to choose between being seen and being myself.

I could be both.

Reflections Pages

1. A moment from this chapter that stood out to me:

2. How this moment connects to my own story, family, or childhood:

3. A belief, habit, or pattern I noticed in myself:

4. A more compassionate or truthful way of seeing this part of my story is:

5. One practical step I want to take this week is:

6. What might get in the way:

7. How I can support myself when it feels hard:

8. A Bible verse this chapter reminds me of and why:

____

____

____

9. A prayer, affirmation, or intention I want to carry forward:

____

____

____

Take what serves you, release what doesn't. Healing and learning are slow, holy work — and you are doing beautifully.

Chapter 3

Love in Layers-Navigating Blended Family Life

"If it is possible, as far as it depends on you, live at peace with everyone."

—Romans 12:18

I met Richard and Anderson long before I realized how much they would change my life. At the time, I was a Realtor, and Richard hired me to sell both his condo and his house. He came as a package deal—with a charming four-year-old son, a pit bull, a shih tzu, and a story I hadn't yet lived but would come to cherish deeply.

Let's face it—divorce is never easy. Add in the emotional gravity of having to share your child, and everything intensifies. In those early days, weekdays away from Anderson were hard for Richard, and weekends away from her son were heartbreaking for his mom, Emily. I don't think she liked me much at first—and honestly, I understood. I was stepping into sacred territory.

At the time, I had a Newfoundland named Kubba—my entire world. I know it's a dog I'm correlating to here, but I tried to imagine someone else being responsible for him, someone I didn't know or trust, and I could feel the ache in my chest. That empathy gave me the grace to see Emily's heart through the tension.

So I asked Richard to create a group text with all three of us. On weekends, Anderson was with us, and I'd send her updates. Not selfies of the two of us—nothing performative—but small, simple snapshots. Anderson eating a chocolate chip banana pancake. Anderson zooming around on his Big Wheel. I wanted her to see that her son was safe. Happy. Loved.

That changed everything.

As a stepmom, you learn quickly where your place is—and what it's not. You learn to understand the heart behind someone's reactions. You recognize that sometimes, even when it's hard, love means putting your own feelings on the back burner for the sake of what's best for the child.

And that became our guiding question: What's best for Anderson?

When we filtered every decision, big or small, through that lens, things became clearer. Not easier, but less chaotic. Less reactive.

There was a moment when Anderson, at just five years old, began calling me "Mudder." I thought it was sweet. Until Emily found out—and her response was raw and emotional. She felt like she was being replaced. Her pain was real, and I took it seriously. I did some digging, not to defend myself but to understand. The research showed that when children form strong bonds with step-parents, especially those present early in life, it's actually very natural for them to use a parent-like name. As long as it's respectful, it shouldn't be corrected.

I gently shared what I had learned with Emily, and after a few days of quiet reflection, she called me and said something I will never forget:

"I had prepared myself for Anderson to have a mean stepmom. I was ready for that—I knew how to handle that. But I never imagined how hard it would be to see that he has the best stepmom in the whole world."

Her words brought me to tears. It was one of the most sincere, vulnerable, and selfless things anyone has ever said to me. In that moment, she showed extraordinary strength—the kind that puts a child's well-being above personal pride. It's rare, and it's brave. I will always be grateful for her grace.

There are so many lessons I've learned through loving Anderson—and one of the most important is that consistency between homes matters. Kids shouldn't have to bounce between two different cultures every week. That emotional whiplash is exhausting. We still don't have it all figured out, but we try. We strive to align our rules, our expectations, and even our routines as much as possible—for his sake.

Anderson, too, is the reason I learned to question the labels placed on children.

Long before we had answers, we had questions. So many questions. It was clear from early on that Anderson wasn't developing quite like other kids. He was gentle, cautious—sometimes to a fault. Playground equipment scared him. He didn't climb into cabinets like toddlers tend to do, and things that usually spark joy in kids, like a swing set or a slide, seemed overwhelming. His fine motor skills were delayed, and academically, he didn't quite move at the pace the world expected of him. And yet, no one could give us a clear reason why.

We pursued testing—places like Brains, and evaluations by multiple specialists. One particularly painful report came back when Anderson was four and a half. It concluded that he couldn't replicate a simple red-green-red pattern using colored blocks. That comment broke both of his parents' hearts.

When Richard told me, I couldn't believe it. I wouldn't believe it—not yet. Having grown up in a world where others constantly defined what I couldn't do, I wasn't about to let that happen to Anderson. So that evening, I sat down with him, and we worked gently, patiently, with the blocks. It took some time and sweet determination, but he got it. I'll never forget the look on Richard's face when I showed him—he was stunned, not because he ever doubted his son, but because the professionals had made them feel so helpless.

What I saw was a boy who could absolutely recognize patterns—patterns in stories, in speech, in puzzles, even in people. He just needed someone to slow down, believe in him, and trust his process.

Still, the evaluations remained inconclusive. Everyone seemed to agree something was different—but no one could name it.

So I dug in. I researched. I read everything I could get my hands on—and eventually, I stumbled upon something called hypotonia. Hypotonia isn't a disease, but a symptom that often points to something deeper. It means the muscles don't have the tone or strength they typically should, which can make a child appear unusually flexible, floppy, or physically weak. It can affect everything from movement and posture to coordination, and it often contributes to developmental delays. When I read the description, it felt like it had been written just for Anderson.

Still, we didn't know what it was a symptom of.

It wasn't until he was seven that a doctor finally ordered an MRI. That scan brought us the answer we'd long been waiting for—Anderson had cerebral palsy.

Getting that diagnosis was a turning point. Not just because it finally gave a name to the mystery, but because it gave us direction. It helped us understand the challenges Anderson had been facing—and just as importantly, how to better support him.

As a family, we had to come together, across two households, to navigate that path. We had to coordinate therapies, follow through on routines, communicate openly, and keep showing up for Anderson with consistency and care. It wasn't always smooth. But it was sacred work.

Loving Anderson has taught me so much—about empathy, about restraint, and about what it truly means to show up for a child with no strings attached.

Loving Anderson shaped the kind of mother I wanted to be—and showed me just how much love my heart could hold. He opened my heart to a love that was bigger than biology. But soon after our wedding, when Richard and I tried to grow our family, we found ourselves on a journey we never could have predicted—one filled with heartbreak, hope, and miracles. And it would be Anderson's faith that would carry us through.

Reflections Pages

1. A moment from this chapter that stood out to me:

2. How this moment connects to my own story, family, or childhood:

3. A belief, habit, or pattern I noticed in myself:

4. A more compassionate or truthful way of seeing this part of my story is:

____

____

____

____

5. One practical step I want to take this week is:

____

____

____

6. What might get in the way:

____

____

____

7. How I can support myself when it feels hard:

____

____

____

8. A Bible verse this chapter reminds me of and why:

____

____

____

9. A prayer, affirmation, or intention I want to carry forward:

____

____

____

Take what serves you, release what doesn't. Healing and learning are slow, holy work — and you are doing beautifully.

Chapter 4

The Road to Motherhood

"I am the Lord, the God of all mankind. Is anything too hard for me?"

—Jeremiah 32:27

Shortly after Richard and I were married, we began talking about growing our family. Anderson, just five at the time, made it clear he was fully on board—he wanted a baby brother or sister. But we quickly discovered that having a child wasn't going to be as easy as we'd hoped.

We started with all the basics—tracking, timing, monitoring—trying to let nature take its course. But months passed with no success. Eventually, we saw a specialist and learned I had a heart-shaped uterus, a condition that made it difficult—if not impossible—for an embryo to properly implant. I underwent surgery to correct it, hopeful that this would solve everything. It didn't.

After more time, more hope, and more disappointment, we moved on to IVF. The clinic we chose was in Chicago, three hours away from our home, which meant that during the weeks of daily blood draws and multiple injections, I stayed alone in a hotel, away from my family. I had a genuine fear of needles, stemming from several traumatic childhood experiences where nurses missed my veins, and many, many blood draws occurred. But I had to overcome that fear—fast. I gave myself 7 to 9 injections a day, all while showing up each morning for more bloodwork.

It was grueling. But it wasn't all bad.

On weekends, Richard and Anderson would make the long drive to come visit me. Anderson, just six at the time, was fascinated by the process. He'd sit beside me, wide-eyed and curious, asking questions as I prepared my injections. He wasn't scared—just sincerely invested. In his own quiet way, he was cheering me on. He even lost his very first tooth during one of those visits, right in the middle of our shared IVF adventure. And in the hotel pool, with no grand plan other than to pass the time together, I had the joy of teaching him how to swim. I still remember his proud little grin as he kicked across the shallow end. Even in the midst of all the fear and grief, there were glimmers of joy. And Anderson was a big part of that.

Our first round of IVF failed. The second, however, was a success—and we were overjoyed. I can still remember the exact feeling: hope blooming like spring after a long winter. But soon my hCG levels plateaued, and we learned that the baby wouldn't make it. I was only six weeks along, but that baby lives forever in my heart. I named him—or her—Christian Rene. Christian, for "follower of Christ." Rene, for "born again."

We grieved, then tried again. The third round failed, but the fourth brought another positive test. This time, we were cautiously hopeful. But joy soon turned to sorrow when we learned the pregnancy was ectopic. The embryo had implanted in my fallopian tube, not my uterus. There was no way for the baby to survive. I was told I had to terminate the pregnancy immediately.

I will never forget that day.

Richard and I arrived at the clinic, faces swollen with tears, hearts heavy with grief. The nurse was cheerful—strangely so—and it felt painfully out of place. I was asked to place my hands on the counter, a blue and gray flecked Formica surface I'll never forget. I watched my tears fall onto it as I received two injections—one in each hip—of a drug that would stop the pregnancy. The same drug used in chemotherapy. It burned going in. But not nearly as much as the ache in my soul.

That night, I broke. I screamed at God. I sobbed with a depth I'd never known. I begged to understand why motherhood came so easily to women who didn't even seem to want it, while I—who longed for it with every fiber of my being—was left empty. That baby, I named Olivia Faith. She was loved. She still is.

We took time to heal. My body needed rest. My spirit even more so. But eventually, we decided to try one last time—mostly because we had a stockpile of unused medication. I remember waking up from the embryo transfer, still groggy from anesthesia, with Richard cracking jokes beside me to make me smile. When the doctor walked in, we dared to hope.

But the look on his face said it all.

With zero bedside manner, he told us the procedure had failed. Not only had it failed, but, in his words, I had failed. "It's your body," he said flatly. "You're broken."

Our hope shattered.

We turned our hearts toward adoption. Anderson, now seven, had faithfully prayed every night for a baby brother or sister in my tummy. But after that final loss, I gently told him that his sibling might come from another woman's tummy. He looked at me, quiet for a moment, then said, "But I want it to come from yours." It broke me—but I didn't stop him from praying that prayer. Night after night, he kept praying. Even when I couldn't.

Three months later, I went in for a routine foot surgery. Just before the IV was placed, a nurse rushed in and stopped the procedure. "You're pregnant," she said.

I laughed. I told her that wasn't possible—that I'd been told, unequivocally, that I could not get pregnant. But the pregnancy test had lit up instantly. Still in disbelief, I asked for a blood draw.

When the results came back, they said my hCG level was 14,001.

I had never gotten above 1,000 before.

We were stunned. Joyful. Terrified. Hopeful. We drove straight to the OB/GYN, and there she was on the ultrasound screen—a tiny 8-week-old bean with a beating heart. Our daughter. Our miracle.

We waited until I was 12 weeks pregnant before telling Anderson. When we finally did, he looked at us and said calmly, "I know." We stared at him, stunned. "How could you know?"

"Because," he said, "that's what I prayed for."

I had lost hope—but Anderson hadn't. And God heard him.

We named her Lucy Fay.

After she was born, our hearts overflowed with gratitude. We wanted to honor God and show our thanks for the miracle He gave us. In a moment that still gives me goosebumps, Richard, Anderson, and I were baptized together—our family, reborn in every sense of the word.

"I am the Lord, the God of all mankind. Is anything too hard for me?" —Jeremiah 32:27

Read that again.

Let it sink in—not as a platitude, but as a promise. That verse isn't poetic fluff. It's the truth. Eternal, immovable truth. And I am living proof that it's real.

There is nothing too hard for Him. Not even this.

We didn't know it then, but Lucy's life was already answering Anderson's prayers—before we ever saw two pink lines. I believe children have an unmatched ability to hear from God, especially when their hearts are open and their prayers are unfiltered. And Anderson's heart was as pure as they come. His unwavering faith gave ours the strength to rise. And when Lucy finally arrived, she became the spark that would light a new way forward—not only for our family, but for everything I thought I knew about education, childhood, and what it means to be seen.

Reflections Pages

1. A moment from this chapter that stood out to me:

2. How this moment connects to my own story, family, or childhood:

3. A belief, habit, or pattern I noticed in myself:

4. A more compassionate or truthful way of seeing this part of my story is:

5. One practical step I want to take this week is:

6. What might get in the way:

7. How I can support myself when it feels hard:

8. A Bible verse this chapter reminds me of and why:

____

____

____

9. A prayer, affirmation, or intention I want to carry forward:

____

____

____

Take what serves you, release what doesn't. Healing and learning are slow, holy work — and you are doing beautifully.

Part 2

The Spark That Lit the Way

These are the stories that ignited everything—where curiosity met calling, and motherhood met mission. From Lucy's earliest learning to the faith that carried us through, this part captures the holy beginnings of a homemade education and the gentle unfolding of a light-filled childhood.

Chapter 5

Rooted in Light: Returning to What Learning Was Meant to Be

"Before I formed you in the womb I knew you, before you were born I set you apart."

—Jeremiah 1:5

By the time I became pregnant with Lucy, I had already begun to see myself differently—not as someone limited by learning challenges, but as someone equipped by them. That shift in perspective changed how I viewed education, potential, and the sacred power of being seen. I didn't want to raise a child who chased perfection. I wanted to raise a child who loved to learn—who felt safe, supported, and full of wonder.

I want to be clear: I don't believe Lucy is "gifted" in the way society defines it. She is not a savant. She didn't come into the world decoding Greek or doing algebra in her sleep. Learning has had its rhythms, and we've had hard days, too. But from the very beginning, Lucy was focused.

Even as a newborn, she locked eyes with people—steady, searching, unafraid. It felt like she was studying the world from the moment she arrived, as if life itself was a great book she couldn't wait to read. That sense of wonder—that deep, holy curiosity—is something all children are born with. My mission was simply to protect it.

From affection to nutrition to environment, I made it my goal to nourish the incredible mind God had entrusted to us. I didn't aim to "get ahead"—I aimed to stay attuned. I gave her a peaceful, predictable rhythm she could count on—not a rigid schedule, but a steady beat that offered both structure and freedom. Our "learning time" became one of the most sacred parts of our day.

At first, that time was mostly spent reading. As soon as she could hold her head up and track movement, I traced words with my finger across the page. That image from To Kill a Mockingbird—of Atticus showing Scout the letters on a newspaper—always stayed with me. It reminded me how important it is to show our children the building blocks, even when they seem too young to understand.

We also used picture cards. I'd lay them out, wait for her to touch one, and name it with joy and animation. "Lucy, that's a dog! Dog says woof woof!" It wasn't about drilling. It was about connection. I wasn't following an age chart—I was following her.

By the time she was just over a year old, Lucy began naming letters. At first, I assumed it was mimicry. But she knew them. She began pointing to letters in books, signs, and packaging—

calling them out with confidence. Her dad and I were stunned. We hadn't set out to teach her the alphabet. We were just creating an environment where learning could blossom naturally.

When she was two, I told her we couldn't stop at a store she liked because I didn't think they're open. She looked out the window, pointed at the glowing neon sign, and said, "That says Open." I was speechless. She was reading.

And it wasn't just letters. Lucy had an early love of numbers, an uncanny sense of geography, and a deep, intuitive hunger for books, conversation, and information. It felt, at times, otherworldly. But I wasn't trying to raise a prodigy. I was just present. I watched. I listened. I gave her time and space, and I met her with joy at every turn.

So when other parents started asking how I "taught her" to read, or how I'd raised such a polite, inquisitive little girl, I often didn't know what to say—because it wasn't just one thing. It was everything.

It was the food she ate and the sugar she didn't.

The books instead of screens.

The hours of unhurried snuggles.

The calm, consistent rhythm of our days.

Everything mattered. And every small choice helped her mind flourish the way God designed it to.

But even deeper than all that, something quieter was guiding me: the way I watched her. The way I trusted her. The way I chose to believe that age wasn't a limitation—and neither was expectation.

I had once been a child who lived under the weight of labels and assumptions. Now I was a mother who could offer something different. Something healing.

Because I had finally learned how to recognize brilliance in places the world doesn't always look.

And that changed everything.

By the time Lucy was three, we had read thousands of pages together—and I don't mean that figuratively. We'd visit the library and fill my biggest tote with as many books as it could hold—usually 22 to 24 titles. Some days, we'd move from one stack to the next, breaking only for snacks, snuggles, or sudden bursts of curiosity that pulled us into spontaneous adventures: tracing the shadow of a wild-looking twig, collecting leaves to identify by their vein patterns, or chasing a butterfly just to see where it would land.

Her questions were relentless in the best possible way:

"Why does the moon follow us?"

"Do clouds get tired?"

"Why do leaves change color?"

I didn't always have the answers, but I always had time. And that time became the soil where Lucy's love of learning took root.

Even as a toddler, her capacity for observation and memory was remarkable. By 14 months, she was helping with simple chores—putting dirty clothes in the hamper, fetching toilet paper from the cabinet, refilling the holder. She could also respond to phonetic cues I built into object associations: "A is for Apple" followed by a crunch sound, or "D is for Duck" followed by a quack. She could identify all 16 picture cards I laid in front of her, toddling over with delight to retrieve the correct one when I asked, "Lucy, can you find the doggy? The doggy goes 'woof woof woof!'"

By 15 months, she was matching objects by color. At 17 months, she began naming complex colors and even crystals—geode, turquoise, rose quartz, jasper, and amethyst. By 18 months, she was pointing at words in books as I read, and she could also play the game Memory with ease. She identified every letter in the alphabet and named dog breeds—Corgi, Poodle, Dalmatian, Shiba Inu—thanks to a dog breed matching game we played. These were milestones most developmental charts place years down the road.

Books were everywhere: on the breakfast table, in the car, in her bed. Screens, on the other hand, were nearly non-existent. We spent our days exploring parks, orchards, zoos, and nature trails. She learned how to be kind to animals—and people—with consistent discipline and gentle guidance. We traveled, too. By age three, Lucy had already visited 15 states and two other countries. The picture cards were great, but nothing compares to the classroom God provides in nature.

I was committed: if I was going to be a stay-at-home mom, then I was going to be fully present—intentional, engaged, and consistent. That meant nurturing, educating, and disciplining with purpose. It wasn't always easy. Some days, I desperately wanted to plop her on the couch with a show just to catch my breath. But I believed God had made me strong enough to handle the hard moments. And I wasn't doing it alone. My husband was my rock—grocery shopping after work, cooking dinner, folding laundry without being asked, showing up without complaint. When I questioned my worth or wondered if I was doing enough, he lifted me up—reminding me that there is no more important work than raising a child, and no better investment than helping Lucy become who she was made to be. He truly valued my role as a mother, and that helped me value it even more.

We always kept puzzles out—everything from chunky toddler boards to 200-piece sets. Lucy chose what looked fun, and we followed her lead. By age two, she was breezing through 100-piece puzzles. One moment I'll never forget was watching her and Richard working on one together. Amazed, he asked, "How can she do puzzles for six-year-olds but still be in diapers?" I gently reminded him that our pediatrician advised us to let her decide when she was ready—or risk a power struggle we'd definitely lose.

One day, as she was placing a puzzle piece, he asked, "Lucy, are you a big girl or a baby?"

"I'm a big girl!" she answered.

"But big girls don't wear diapers," he said.

(I shot him a playful glare from the kitchen—classic Dad move.)

Without missing a beat, Lucy pressed the puzzle piece into place and replied, "Well, babies can't talk."

Checkmate. Toddler style.

Again, I don't think Lucy is a genius. I think she's a joyful learner who's been given space, exposure, and the tools to thrive. And I believe—truly—that many children could reach unexpected heights if we simply gave them time, attention, and trust.

By the time Lucy was nearly three, it was clear she was ready for more.

In June of 2022, I ordered a collection of learning tools and books from The Good and the Beautiful homeschool program. Around that same time, we also enrolled her in a local nature-based outdoor school, where she attended three half-days a week. Over the next two years, this gave her more than just fresh air and muddy boots—it nurtured a deep love for the natural world and offered meaningful opportunities to grow socially.

In August of 2023, we began the Preschool Course Set at home. Lucy thrived. She zipped through the material with joy and curiosity. By April 2024, she had started Kindergarten-level math and language arts. I supplemented with the Little Hearts and Hands science program—story-based, beautifully illustrated, and perfectly suited to her age.

We began slowly, just one lesson in each subject per day. But that pace didn't last long. Lucy began asking for two lessons a day, and by summer, she had completed the entire Kindergarten level and moved into first grade.

To be clear: I wasn't trying to accelerate her through childhood. There's so much more to life than bookwork, and I cherish the richness of unstructured time. But I wanted to honor her pace. Two lessons each of math and language arts may sound intense, but at this stage, our school time rarely lasted more than 90 minutes. The rest of our day was filled with movement, laughter, nature, and wonder.

I never skipped lessons—each one laid an important foundation. But I did make thoughtful accommodations. If something came easily, I shortened the practice. If writing became tiring, I'd step in as her scribe. Small adjustments kept learning joyful, and they made all the difference.

Reflections Pages

1. A moment from this chapter that stood out to me:

2. How this moment connects to my own story, family, or childhood:

3. A belief, habit, or pattern I noticed in myself:

4. A more compassionate or truthful way of seeing this part of my story is:

5. One practical step I want to take this week is:

6. What might get in the way:

7. How I can support myself when it feels hard:

8. A Bible verse this chapter reminds me of and why:

____

____

____

9. A prayer, affirmation, or intention I want to carry forward:

____

____

____

Take what serves you, release what doesn't. Healing and learning are slow, holy work — and you are doing beautifully.

Chapter 6

A Light That Fits: Honoring the Unique Way Every Child Learns

"Train up a child in the way he should go; even when he is old he will not depart from it."

—Proverbs 22:6

There comes a moment in every parent's journey when you realize that love alone isn't enough—you also need a plan. By the time Lucy was five, it was clear we needed to make an intentional decision about what kind of education would best serve her heart, her mind, and her spirit. Traditional school? Homeschooling? Something in between?

Richard and I spent many long conversations weighing our options. We knew Lucy needed academic freedom. She was already working through material far beyond her age, and we didn't want her held back simply because of the year she was born. At the same time, we deeply valued the social experiences that come with a classroom—learning to work with peers, handle conflict, play games at recess, and participate in school traditions. But the thought of her attending class alongside much older children didn't sit right either.

It was a real tension—one that tugged at our hearts in both directions. We prayed about it. We talked to friends and mentors. And then, one afternoon, we stumbled across a local Christian school offering a Homeschool Connection Program: one day a week, children could attend in-person classes with peers their own age, while continuing core subjects at home. They'd enjoy specials like music, Spanish, gym, and art—all the "extras" that often get lost in homeschool curricula. As we read the description, our hearts stirred. This wasn't just a solution. It was an answered prayer.

We enrolled Lucy immediately.

The program met every Wednesday. From the very first day, Lucy was hooked. She had her own little backpack, her first lunchbox, and an outfit she'd picked out with careful pride. I think I was more nervous than she was. Would she feel out of place? Would she make friends? Would her teachers understand her unique learning pace and needs?

Each week, she came home with stories—about the games they played in gym, the Spanish words they sang in circle time, the friendships she was forming, the art projects still drying in her cubby. She was thriving—not just academically, but socially, emotionally, and spiritually.

Back at home, our rhythms continued: our cozy morning routines, our nature walks, our puzzles on the floor. But now, Wednesdays had become something sacred. They brought structure, excitement, and community—not just for Lucy, but for me too. I began to savor the quiet hours while she was at school—time to plan, recharge, or simply breathe. It became a beautiful rhythm.

She didn't have to miss out on treasured childhood milestones—Valentine's Day card exchanges, Christmas concerts, birthday celebrations, or giggling with friends at recess. That was one of the greatest blessings of the Homeschool Connection Program. Every Wednesday, Lucy stepped into a classroom filled with art supplies, musical instruments, and the joyful chaos of childhood. She got to hang her backpack on a hook, pass out homemade Valentines, sing in the Christmas program, and run across the playground with kids her age. It was the balance we'd prayed for—an answer that blended the best of both worlds.

There were still hard days. After the "honeymoon period" wore off, Lucy went through a stretch of tearful drop-offs that lasted a few weeks. Not loud, wailing sobs—but soft, heartbreaking tears. The kind that makes you question everything. I'd crouch down, stroke her back, whisper encouragements, and remind her she was brave. But once I walked back to the car, I'd sit in the driver's seat with my own eyes full of tears.

Was I making her too attached by homeschooling her? Or worse—was I pushing her out of the nest too soon? Those thoughts swirled in opposite directions, each with its own weight. That's the torment of a mom's mind sometimes—wondering if every choice is either too much or not enough.

But week by week, the tears faded. And in their place came confidence, stories, and joy. And in my place at the curb stood a little girl who ran into the building with a smile.

Lucy also began forming real, lasting friendships. The school organized a trip to a local nursing home, where the children made crafts with residents, listened to their stories, and sang songs together. My heart soared watching her develop not only social skills, but compassion and empathy. She was blooming.

As time passed, I realized something profound: this hybrid path we'd chosen wasn't a compromise. It was a gift. Lucy had space to soar in her learning without pressure or burnout. She had a community of peers, kindhearted teachers, and meaningful experiences. And I had the privilege of walking beside her—not just as her mom, but as her teacher, her cheerleader, her witness.

Something else happened during those quiet Wednesday hours—something I didn't expect. I found pieces of myself again. With Lucy at school for the day, I had a sliver of silence. Stillness. Space. And in that space, I could plan, tidy, pray, write, or just sit with a cup of coffee and remember who I was beyond the role of "Mom."

It reminded me that I wasn't just pouring into Lucy—I was still a person in need of refilling, too. And far from being selfish, that space made me a more grounded, joyful, and attentive teacher the rest of the week.

This journey of educational intention didn't just shape Lucy—it reshaped how we approached learning as a family. We began to see that traditional paths don't always serve every child equally. Around the same time, we were watching Anderson struggle in the public school system. He was bright, inquisitive, and full of insight, but it wasn't being reflected in his progress reports. Teachers marked concepts as "mastered" when, clearly, they weren't. It was frustrating—and heartbreaking—for all of us.

After a lot of discussion, collaboration, and prayer between our homes, we found an incredible charter school near where Anderson lives with his mom. One of the things that drew us in was its mastery-based model: students must score at least 80% before moving on to new material. If they fall short, they revisit what they missed and retest—ensuring real understanding before advancement. It felt like such a respectful, empowering approach to learning—one that gives children the time and support they need. And it was a much better fit for Anderson.

Seeing both of our children flourish in environments tailored to their needs confirmed something I've come to believe with my whole heart: children aren't cookie cutters. They are handcrafted by God, each with its own rhythm, its own needs, and its own potential. And as parents, our job isn't to mold them into a system. It's to build a system that honors who they already are.

It wasn't always easy. There were days of doubt, moments of exhaustion, and times I questioned if we were doing it "right." But in those moments, I'd look at our kids—curled up with a book, asking thoughtful questions, telling jokes at dinner—and I'd remember: they weren't meant to be crammed into someone else's mold. They were made to shine in their own way.

And somehow, by God's grace, we're giving them space to do just that.

Reflections Pages

1. A moment from this chapter that stood out to me:

2. How this moment connects to my own story, family, or childhood:

3. A belief, habit, or pattern I noticed in myself:

4. A more compassionate or truthful way of seeing this part of my story is:

5. One practical step I want to take this week is:

6. What might get in the way:

7. How I can support myself when it feels hard:

8. A Bible verse this chapter reminds me of and why:

____

____

____

9. A prayer, affirmation, or intention I want to carry forward:

____

____

____

Take what serves you, release what doesn't. Healing and learning are slow, holy work — and you are doing beautifully.

Chapter 7

Letting Curiosity Lead

"Whatever you do, do it all for the glory of God."

—1 Corinthians 10:31

Homeschooling, for us, has never been about recreating a classroom at the kitchen table. Parts of our day reflect that—structured lessons, books spread across the counter—but the heart of our learning is something softer, deeper. It's about listening—to Lucy's questions, her rhythms, her spark—and letting that lead the way.

Some mornings begin with books. Others, with bugs. One day might open with subtraction and journal prompts; the next, with a field trip to a science museum or a deep dive into why clouds look the way they do. (Cue the crayons, scissors, and overflowing paint palette.) The beauty of this season is not just the flexibility in our schedule, but the freedom to let curiosity shape the curriculum.

And here's what I want to say loud and clear: you don't have to homeschool to follow your child's curiosity. You don't have to throw out structure to make space for wonder. Whether your child is at home, in public school, private school, or anything in between, there's value in paying close attention. Curiosity is a flame. It can be fanned no matter where your child learns.

Anderson is a perfect example of that. Though his educational path is more traditional, we've worked hard—together with his mom—to ensure it's still curiosity-led and rooted in what lights him up. One of Anderson's greatest loves is football. He can tell you the stats of every player on his favorite teams, recite plays, and recount game highlights like he was born to be a sportscaster. The boy who was once labeled as having trouble retaining information could recall every detail from last night's game without missing a beat. So we used that passion as a bridge—channeling his reading through sports biographies, game-day recaps, and play-by-play books that made reading feel exciting and personal. Emily even took him to live games, where the whole experience became a living classroom. That's the secret, really: you just have to find the spark—and fan it.

Because of the flexibility in our days, we've also been able to explore all kinds of activities—each one offering something different for the body, mind, or heart. Gymnastics built balance and body awareness. Karate introduced discipline and self-defense (ahya!). Dance invited grace and poise—complete with slippers and a tutu, of course. Swimming was non-negotiable—a life skill we took seriously. Tennis? Why not! Music and art? Always worth a try. Not every activity will become a long-term passion, and that was never the goal. Each one is an invitation—a chance for Lucy to stretch, grow, and discover what made her come alive.

Some things would stick. Others wouldn't. But for us, that isn't failure—it's feedback. Each experience brought new lessons: resilience, confidence, humility, and joy. And it reminded Lucy (and me) that learning doesn't only happen at a desk. It happens in gyms, on stages, in pools, on courts, in the rhythm of movement and music, through trial and triumph.

I loved watching Lucy's growth through these experiences. When she first began karate, gymnastics, and dance at age three, she was incredibly shy. If she didn't understand something, she'd tear up—overwhelmed by the unfamiliar. But her instructors were patient, nurturing, and wise. Over time, her confidence began to bloom.

I'll never forget the day she had a karate tournament in the morning and a dance recital in the afternoon. And I do mean immediately after—she was literally transforming from a ninja to a ballerina in the backseat of our car. I watched in awe as she delivered her karate forms—one with a weapon, one without—with strength and poise. Just a year earlier, this same tournament had her in tears for weeks leading up to it. She'd rushed through her routine just to get it over with. But not this time. This time, the little warrior owned it.

Then we zipped across town to her recital. Same girl, different shoes. I watched her float across the stage—graceful, radiant, composed. It wasn't just a costume change; it was a deep understanding of presence. She knew how to bring fierceness when it was time to fight, and softness when it was time to dance.

Exposing her to such different activities was proving to be more meaningful than I ever anticipated. They weren't just teaching her physical skills—they were shaping her inner world, helping her embody the emotions, character traits, and confidence that came with each role. And as I watched it all unfold before my eyes, I was completely in awe.

Watching that transformation made me reflect on how we choose the activities she participates in—and why.

I always made her finish what she started. That was non-negotiable. But within that framework, I gave her space to grow, change, and decide what was worth continuing. And while some activities came and went, others became part of her foundation. Swimming and karate, for example, are priorities in our home—non-negotiables that we commit to deeply.

We also take time to understand animals. Beyond the local zoo, I sign Lucy up for classes at a nearby farm where she learns to be gentle with baby chicks and assertive while walking goats. These experiences teach such valuable lessons—ones that help shape the fabric of character and compassion.

Anderson, too, has had his share of curiosity-driven moments—like the time he spent hours practicing a specific football throw he read about in a book, determined to get it just right. On the weekend, he and Lucy devoted themselves to building a cushion fort that could withstand both the cats' sneak attacks and the dogs' full-speed barreling. Whether in a classroom or in the chaos of a weekend at home, learning is always happening if you're watching for it.

And we're still exploring. I haven't yet found the right musical outlet for Lucy, but I'm always on the lookout. She belts out lyrics in the car with such confidence and conviction, I know there's something stirring beneath the surface—some musical thread waiting to be tugged. Maybe it's voice lessons. Maybe piano. Maybe something we haven't even thought of yet.

Anderson, too, is discovering where his passions lie. He's recently taken an interest in weightlifting—asking questions, watching videos, and trying out exercises with Richard. He's also developed a love for cooking, often jumping in to help with meals or experimenting in the kitchen with creativity and focus. Just like with Lucy, we're paying attention—listening for those sparks of curiosity that might grow into something more.

Isn't that the way of parenthood? Always wondering if you're doing enough or too much, if you're guiding or rushing, planting seeds or pushing the soil too soon. I've learned to live in the wonder of it—trusting that curiosity will show us the way.

And when it does, we try to follow. Whether it's a weekend pottery class, a nature walk after dinner, or a new instrument just waiting to be strummed, saying yes to those sparks—big or small—brings a kind of fullness that's rooted in connection, intention, and joy. It doesn't have to be all day or every day. It just has to be noticed.

This chapter of life is messy, beautiful, and gloriously unscripted. But one thing I've learned for sure: when you let curiosity lead, wonder always follows.

Find that spark—and start fanning.

Reflections Pages

1. A moment from this chapter that stood out to me:

____

____

____

2. How this moment connects to my own story, family, or childhood:

____

____

____

3. A belief, habit, or pattern I noticed in myself:

____

____

____

4. A more compassionate or truthful way of seeing this part of my story is:

____

5. One practical step I want to take this week is:

6. What might get in the way:

7. How I can support myself when it feels hard:

8. A Bible verse this chapter reminds me of and why:

____

____

____

9. A prayer, affirmation, or intention I want to carry forward:

____

____

____

Take what serves you, release what doesn't. Healing and learning are slow, holy work — and you are doing beautifully.

Chapter 8

Faith & Family - A Home Rooted in Both

"But as for me and my household, we will serve the Lord."

—Joshua 24:15

It started with a cappuccino and a Bible podcast.

After Lucy was born and we made the decision to homeschool, our hearts were not just focused on her education—we were focused on the kind of home we wanted to build. And for Richard and me, that meant returning to our roots and rediscovering the faith that had quietly threaded through our lives but hadn't always taken center stage.

I was raised attending Christian school, memorizing verses and walking through the stories of the Bible as a student rather than a seeker. I even traveled to Israel, touching the places where miracles once walked. I believed in God. But I didn't yet know Him.

When Richard and I got married, faith was present, but inconsistent. We said grace at meals, talked about our values, and felt the tug of spiritual truth—but we weren't anchored yet. Then came the trying seasons of infertility, IVF, and miscarriage. And as so many people of faith know, hardship can harden you, or it can hollow you out just enough for God to pour in something new.

After Lucy was born—and especially after our family baptism—something shifted. We wanted more than lukewarm faith. We wanted to live like people who believed the Bible was true. So we started listening to The Bible Recap by Tara-Leigh Cobble every morning as we worked out together in our home gym. The format—a short daily reading followed by a 7- to 10-minute recap—was easy to digest and easy to stick with.

But it did something unexpected. It didn't just educate us. It transformed us.

For the first time, the Bible wasn't just a historical text. It was a living conversation. We found ourselves pausing the podcast, asking questions, diving deeper, and carrying those conversations into breakfast with the kids. We began noticing how our perspective on everything shifted—parenting, marriage, work, even rest. Our hearts softened. Our awareness grew. Our desire to walk with God wasn't a checkbox anymore. It became the quiet pulse of our home.

I noticed it changing Lucy's life first. Children are far more spiritually attuned than we often realize. She started asking deep questions, drawing pictures of Bible stories, and even pretending to "teach" Sunday School to her stuffed animals. On car rides, she'd say things like, "Mom, did you notice the clouds God made for you today?"—a nod to how we've taught our kids to see beauty as a gift from God, little moments He places in our path to make us smile. At bedtime, she'd often ask, "Can we talk to Jesus together?" And during quiet moments in the middle of the day, I'd catch her humming worship songs while doing puzzles or coloring—her faith woven gently into the rhythm of her play.

Anderson took it in differently. His spiritual journey has always been quieter, more private—but the reverence is unmistakable. Sometimes he'll ask theological questions that make us pause and wonder, "How did you even think of that?" His faith is steady, thoughtful, and sincere. The kind that sticks because it's personal.

That's what we hope for both of them. Not religion for the sake of structure, but relationship for the sake of life.

We don't claim to have all the answers. We still have hard days, distracted mornings, and moments where our faith feels less like a fire and more like a flicker. But we return to the flame. And we show our kids how to return to it, too.

Because raising children in the light doesn't mean keeping them from the dark, it means teaching them where to find the Source when the darkness comes.

Faith gave us our foundation—but learning is where our days took shape. As our home became more deeply rooted in both love and truth, I began to see just how connected the two were. Educating our kids wasn't just about academics; it was about nurturing a whole child—heart, mind, and soul.

This foundation didn't make the journey easier, but it made it meaningful. It gave us something to come back to—again and again—as we walked through the moments that would shape us.

Reflections Pages

1. A moment from this chapter that stood out to me:

2. How this moment connects to my own story, family, or childhood:

3. A belief, habit, or pattern I noticed in myself:

4. A more compassionate or truthful way of seeing this part of my story is:

5. One practical step I want to take this week is:

6. What might get in the way:

7. How I can support myself when it feels hard:

8. A Bible verse this chapter reminds me of and why:

____

____

____

9. A prayer, affirmation, or intention I want to carry forward:

____

____

____

Take what serves you, release what doesn't. Healing and learning are slow, holy work — and you are doing beautifully.

Part 3: Formed by the Moments

Character isn't built in a vacuum—it's shaped in the real, often messy moments of growing up. This part explores what children learn when they face hard things, make mistakes, ask big questions, and stretch into who they're becoming. It's about math meltdowns and playground politics, deep breaths and do-overs—and the quiet beauty of standing tall, even when standing corrected.

Chapter 9

Math without Tears

"Whatever you do, work at it with all your heart, as working for the Lord, not for human masters."

—Colossians 3:23

There's a common misconception that early readers are automatically "gifted" in all subjects. Spoiler alert: they're not. Just because Lucy could devour a chapter book before age five didn't mean she could easily navigate the language of numbers. In fact, her rapid advancement in reading made math feel all the more humbling—for both of us.

It wasn't that she couldn't do math. She absolutely could. It was that math didn't come with the same natural ease as literature or language arts. And for a child so used to things clicking quickly, anything that required repetition and effort felt foreign. Frustrating. Sometimes, it is even defeating. I had to learn to tread carefully—neither shielding her from hard things nor making them feel like punishment. It was a delicate balance, especially for someone like me who was once traumatized by traditional math instruction myself.

And I say that not only as a mother, but as someone who grew up with a learning disability. School often felt like a place where I was measured by everything I couldn't do, rather than the strengths I hadn't yet discovered. The label of "disabled" weighed heavily, even though the truth was, I simply learned differently. I still do.

So, when I sit with my daughter during a tough math lesson, I carry all of that with me. I know what it feels like to struggle, to be misunderstood, to wonder if you'll ever get there. I know how rare and sacred this moment is—even the hard parts. Especially the hard parts. Because they mean she's here. And she's learning.

And even when something didn't come naturally to Lucy, we didn't quit. We just found a new path.

That's one of the many reasons I'm so grateful to homeschool Lucy. Knowing her deep love for stories, I've been able to tailor her education to fit the way she learns best. I found a math program rooted in language and storytelling—not because it's "easier," but because it's richer. It doesn't just drill facts; it weaves them into meaningful narratives. It doesn't simply seek answers; it invites curiosity. Math becomes more than numbers—it becomes a lens through which she can explore people, patterns, cultures, and connection. And perhaps most importantly, it doesn't expect the child to mold to the lesson—it allows the lesson to gently mold to the child.

Learning styles vary as wildly as personalities—and that's something to embrace, not erase.

Take Lucy's current math level, for example—Level 3. With each unit, she follows the journey of a fictional family from a different part of the world. In China, she met Bo and Chun, and while learning place value, she also explored the beauty of Chinese mountains, currency, and food. Then came Winnie and Tombe from Africa, who helped teach geometry and measurement while introducing African traditions and everyday life. We traveled to Quebec, where she practiced metric conversions while mentally tasting maple-syrup-laced dishes. Then to New Delhi, India, where fractions came alive in the kitchen and math became a passport to the world.

For Lucy, that story-based structure is magic. It anchors her learning in meaning. She remembers what she's learned—not because she's drilled with flashcards, but because she makes connections. Her education isn't a patchwork of disconnected facts. It's a tapestry—stitched with context, curiosity, and joy. Again, it's all about finding that spark!

However, that kind of learning wouldn't work for every child. It certainly wouldn't be the best fit for Anderson. For him, too many layers in a lesson can make the core concept harder to find. He thrives on clarity, on simplicity, on information that is structured and direct. Lucy thrives on wonder and narrative. And both are right. Both are valid. The beauty of individualized education is recognizing these differences—not trying to force one method to work for everyone, but instead, finding the approach that fits each child's needs and strengths.

Anderson once told me more football facts than I thought a human brain could hold. I'm talking rosters, stats, game plays, positions, the history of certain teams—you name it. And it hit me: this is how his mind works. When he's captivated by a subject, the information sticks like Velcro. So we used it. I started channeling his learning through that lens—books about sports, writing prompts about athletes, math problems using football scores and statistics. His mom, Emily, would even take him to games, where the sights, sounds, and pacing helped fuel his passion. That so-called "disability" that supposedly made it hard for him to retain information? Turns out, it just depended on the information.

That was a pivotal realization for me: every child has a spark. You just have to find it—and then fan it.

And Lucy's spark? It's connection. If it feels relational, she's all in. That's why math wrapped in story works. It invites her in, gives her a reason to care, and makes hard things feel possible—even enjoyable.

She's still hit milestone after milestone "ahead of schedule"—but not because she's some kind of prodigy. She's not. She's a bright, curious, deeply loved child whose mom simply watches, listens, and responds. I don't force her to do things she's not ready for—but I also don't lower the bar just to make things easier. I set it just high enough for her to stretch, and I let her know I believe she can reach it. That belief—hers and mine—makes all the difference.

As Lucy's academic journey began to unfold, so did another essential layer of her development—the social one. Because as much as we value knowledge, we know that true growth doesn't happen in isolation. It happens in community, in connection, and in those messy, beautiful moments of learning how to live—and love—alongside others.

Reflections Pages

1. A moment from this chapter that stood out to me:

____

____

____

2. How this moment connects to my own story, family, or childhood:

____

____

____

3. A belief, habit, or pattern I noticed in myself:

____

____

____

4. A more compassionate or truthful way of seeing this part of my story is:

____

____

____

____

5. One practical step I want to take this week is:

____

____

____

6. What might get in the way:

____

____

____

7. How I can support myself when it feels hard:

____

____

____

8. A Bible verse this chapter reminds me of and why:

____

____

____

9. A prayer, affirmation, or intention I want to carry forward:

____

____

____

Take what serves you, release what doesn't. Healing and learning are slow, holy work — and you are doing beautifully.

Chapter 10

Social Myths and Real-Life Friends

"A friend loves at all times, and a brother is born for a time of adversity."

—Proverbs 17:17

One of the most persistent misconceptions about homeschooling is that homeschooled kids aren't "socialized." The word itself gets tossed around like some kind of academic vitamin—one that traditional schools supposedly provide in abundance while homeschoolers are left malnourished and awkward. It's the question every homeschool parent hears, and the assumption behind it is almost always the same: But how will your child make friends? As if children can't possibly learn to interact with others unless they're in a crowded classroom five days a week. It always made me smile a little. Lucy, who strikes up conversations in grocery store lines and makes best friends at restaurants, is one of the most social kids I know.

I get it. I really do. Before we started homeschooling, I had that question myself. But now, I can say with complete confidence: not only is Lucy well-socialized—she's thriving socially. And it's not because we've gone out of our way to manufacture some picture-perfect friend group. It's because meaningful friendships are built on far more than shared desks and daily bell schedules. They're built on shared experiences, shared values, and opportunities for connection that feel real—not forced.

Our enrollment in the Homeschool Connection Program has been a huge gift. Once a week, Lucy attends class with peers her own age. They do art projects, gym class, music, and Spanish together. They pass out Valentins, sing in the Christmas concert, and chase each other across the playground. She's not missing out on recess or birthday parties. She's right in the thick of it, building friendships the same way any other child would—by showing up, being herself, and having regular opportunities to play and connect.

One of the unexpected gifts of Lucy's weekly hybrid program and extracurriculars—like karate and playdates—is that they give her a space to navigate friendships, handle conflicts, and even get bossed around by a four-year-old or two. And honestly, those are some of the best life lessons there are.

But here's what I think is even more important: we haven't taught Lucy to fear strangers. We've taught her to discern. There's a difference.

Just last night, we were having dinner at a restaurant with an outdoor patio that overlooked a golf course. There was a patch of open grass nearby where a few kids were twirling and cartwheeling in the golden light of evening. Lucy watched them for a few moments and then turned to me with hopeful eyes, "Mom, can I go play with them after I finish eating?"

I said yes—and in the span of three bites, Lucy had vacuumed up the rest of her dinner. Before I knew it, she was out there laughing, chasing, and skipping with two little girls she had never met before. From strangers to kindred spirits in minutes. Watching her reminded me of something important: connection doesn't require years of history. Sometimes, it only takes openness.

We don't stifle those instincts. We guide them. We teach Lucy what safe boundaries look like, but we also give her the freedom to approach the world with curiosity and confidence.

And while Lucy spends most of her time around family, mentors, and a curated circle of peers, Anderson's social experience has looked quite different. As a child in a traditional school setting, he is surrounded by peer influence nearly every moment of the day. And that has its own learning curve.

Like most kids, Anderson wants to fit in. He wants to belong. And there was a season when that desire made it especially hard for him to stand apart. Many of his classmates were spending hours after school gaming—something we've never prioritized in our home. Anderson knew our values, and for a while, he respected them. But the social pressure eventually crept in. He started sneaking extra gaming time and, even harder for us to face, started lying about whether his schoolwork was done.

It wasn't like him. Anderson had never been dishonest with us before, so we didn't check up on his assignments. We believed him. And his lie worked—for a little while. But eventually, we discovered just how far behind he had fallen. It was a hard moment for all of us. But it became a turning point.

Together—with love and firmness—we got him back on track. And through that experience, Anderson learned about accountability, the consequences of compromise, and the courage it takes to come clean and start again. It reminded us that social environments of any kind come with both positive and negative influences. No system—homeschool, public school, private school—is immune to that. What matters is how we as parents respond. How we course-correct with grace. How we use those hard moments to build trust, not tear it down.

It also reminded me that we're all doing our best with the context we've been given. There's no perfect formula. There's just intentional parenting—and lots of prayer.

I used to feel the sting of skeptical comments:

"Don't you worry, she won't learn to work with others?"

"Aren't you afraid she'll be too sheltered?"

"You know… she needs real-world experiences."

I let those roll off now. Not because I don't care—but because I do. I care enough to trust what I see. I care enough to know that raising kind, discerning, grounded children takes more than proximity to peers. It takes vision. It takes involvement. It takes being the kind of parent who doesn't just ask "who are their friends?"—but also, "who are they becoming?"

Lucy isn't just learning how to coexist—she's learning how to be kind, how to be inclusive, how to hold her own, and how to form genuine friendships in a wide variety of settings. And Anderson, in his own way, is learning those lessons too—sometimes through joyful friendships, sometimes through painful pressures. And through it all, we are walking beside them both.

If that's not real socialization, I don't know what is.

Whether on the playground, in the classroom, or at home, our children are always learning—not just from books, but from each experience, each challenge, each moment of connection. And sometimes, the most powerful lessons don't come from structured environments at all, but from the wild and wonderful spaces where imagination runs free.

Reflections Pages

1. A moment from this chapter that stood out to me:

____

____

____

2. How this moment connects to my own story, family, or childhood:

____

____

____

3. A belief, habit, or pattern I noticed in myself:

____

____

____

4. A more compassionate or truthful way of seeing this part of my story is:

5. One practical step I want to take this week is:

6. What might get in the way:

7. How I can support myself when it feels hard:

8. A Bible verse this chapter reminds me of and why:

____

____

____

9. A prayer, affirmation, or intention I want to carry forward:

____

____

____

Take what serves you, release what doesn't. Healing and learning are slow, holy work — and you are doing beautifully.

Chapter 11

Standing Strong, Standing Corrected

"Be completely humble and gentle; be patient, bearing with one another in love."

—Ephesians 4:2

There's something no one tells you about parenting: you won't always recognize the moment when your child is learning one of life's most important lessons. Sometimes it happens in a classroom or over dinner, but more often, it happens in those raw, unscripted pockets of childhood—on a playground, in a group of peers, during the awkward lull of a conversation. And if you're too quick to step in, you might just rob them of the lesson altogether.

True social growth doesn't only happen in classrooms. It happens wherever kids are given the chance to interact, mess up, reflect, and try again. For Lucy, those chances come in many forms—through playdates, enrichment classes, her one-day-a-week school program, church, extracurriculars, and spontaneous playground friendships. Each interaction becomes part of the invisible curriculum of growing up—and some of the biggest lessons happen when things don't go smoothly.

One moment stands out so clearly that it inspired a picture book of its own.

One afternoon during gymnastics, Lucy joined a small group of girls chatting while they waited for their turn on the high bar. The conversation was light—sharing about activities they did outside of class like dance, swimming, and gymnastics. Lucy, always excited to connect, chimed in that she was in karate and that she was homeschooled. But instead of being met with curiosity or encouragement, the girls stared at her and started to giggle.

They told her they didn't believe her. One began to quiz her with basic math facts, challenging her answers and scoffing when she mentioned she was already learning multiplication. Lucy wasn't trying to boast—she just wanted to be included and believed. But her confidence deflated. One of the older girls, who clearly wasn't familiar with multiplication yet, crossed her arms and walked away in frustration, leaving Lucy confused and heartbroken.

That night at home, the frustration bubbled up. Lucy was angry, and rightfully so. She wanted to say something back—something sharp, something that would've "put them in their place." And honestly, I understood the feeling. But instead of fueling her fire, we helped her process it with grace.

We reminded her that meanness often tries to make others mean too—and that real strength is choosing kindness, even when it's not returned. When you're rooted in who you are, you don't need everyone else's validation to stand tall. And in true dad fashion, Richard leaned in and joked, "A roundhouse kick to one of their tushes would've shown them you're in karate!" That, of course, got the biggest laugh of the evening. The laughter softened the sting. It gave Lucy space to reframe the experience—not as a wound to carry, but as a moment to grow from.

She learned that standing strong doesn't mean fighting back with the same energy you were given. Sometimes it means standing in the truth of who you are, even if others don't recognize it.

But not every social moment casts our children as the hero. Sometimes, they're the ones who need correcting.

There was a playdate when Lucy got upset because a game wasn't going her way. She crossed her arms, scowled, and stomped off, refusing to play at all. Her friend looked hurt and confused. I watched from the sidelines, heart aching, but I didn't jump in. Instead, I let the discomfort linger—because that's where growth begins.

Later, we talked it through. Lucy was teary and embarrassed. "I was just so frustrated," she said. "I didn't mean to be mean."

"I know," I told her. "But feelings don't excuse behavior. When we act out of frustration, we sometimes hurt people we care about. And if we don't face that, we don't grow."

That moment mattered. She apologized to her friend the next time they played. A small thing, maybe. But I could see the roots of maturity taking hold.

Anderson has had his own version of this, too—his wasn't rooted in play or peer conflict, but in the quiet, personal challenge of responsibility.

When he was twelve, Anderson had a major growth spurt. His muscles, already affected by cerebral palsy and the symptom of hypotonia, began to tighten rapidly—so much so that his heels were being pulled off the ground when he walked. The doctors recommended a treatment involving walking casts. For eight weeks, Anderson went in weekly for new casts that gently stretched the muscles in his calves and feet a little more each time. He thought the whole thing was pretty cool—and honestly, he handled it like a champ.

But once the casts came off, a new routine had to begin: daily stretching. It wasn't optional. His doctors made it clear—this would need to become as regular and essential as brushing his teeth for the rest of his life. To help him build consistency and strength, both his mom's home and ours bought identical ellipticals so he could do light cardio and stay flexible. It was all set up for success.

While he was with us, we worked out together and could track his efforts firsthand. But when he was at his mom's house, he assured everyone that he was keeping up with his stretches and workouts.

Only… he wasn't.

The truth came out slowly—through tight muscles, visible discomfort, and eventually an admission. He hadn't been telling the truth. Not because he didn't care, but because—like most preteens—he didn't want to do it. It was boring. It was inconvenient. And he didn't want to be the only one in his friend group who had this kind of responsibility.

So we regrouped. Together, across both homes, we created a new system of accountability. Anderson would send screenshots of his elliptical workouts. We'd check in more consistently and kindly hold him to the standard—not out of punishment, but out of love.

Through that process, he learned something essential: discipline doesn't always feel good in the moment—but it's what allows us to stand tall in the long run. And accountability isn't about control—it's about care.

As parents, it's tempting to fix things, smooth things over, or defend our child's actions. But doing so can rob them of the consequences that teach. If we always rescue them from discomfort, they may never learn the strength that's forged through it.

Whether it's structured play in classes like karate or gymnastics, or everyday responsibilities like medical routines and fitness goals, these moments matter. They teach emotional intelligence, empathy, humility, confidence, and courage.

In gymnastics, Lucy learned how to stand firm—not just in her stances, but in her spirit. It wasn't about physical strength; it was about integrity, self-control, and courage when no one else was watching. These lessons didn't just build her physical confidence; they shaped her character from the inside out.

Both Lucy and Anderson are learning that not everyone will be kind—and sometimes, they won't be either. But each time, they get another chance to try again. To forgive, to be forgiven, and to grow stronger.

Socialization, it turns out, isn't just about being around other kids. It's about becoming the kind of person who treats others well—and knowing how to bounce back when you don't.

So no, Lucy doesn't spend her days in a traditional classroom. But both she and Anderson are learning the lessons that matter most.

They're learning to stand strong.

And just as importantly, they're learning to stand corrected.

But strength isn't only shaped in moments of tension—it's also grown in spaces of freedom and play. And for us, that often begins when we step outside.

Reflections Pages

1. A moment from this chapter that stood out to me:

2. How this moment connects to my own story, family, or childhood:

3. A belief, habit, or pattern I noticed in myself:

4. A more compassionate or truthful way of seeing this part of my story is:

____

____

____

____

5. One practical step I want to take this week is:

____

____

____

6. What might get in the way:

____

____

____

7. How I can support myself when it feels hard:

____

____

____

8. A Bible verse this chapter reminds me of and why:

____

____

____

9. A prayer, affirmation, or intention I want to carry forward:

____

____

____

Take what serves you, release what doesn't. Healing and learning are slow, holy work — and you are doing beautifully.

Chapter 12

Learning in the Wild / The Power of Play

"For since the creation of the world God's invisible qualities… have been clearly seen, being understood from what has been made."

—Romans 1:20

There's something sacred about stepping outside. No matter the mood we're in or the day we've had, the moment our feet hit the grass and our eyes meet the sky, something inside us resets. The air feels different, softer. Quieter. Slower. And somehow, truer.

Nature has become one of our greatest teachers.

Lucy never goes on a walk without a bag—or two. She insists on having something to collect her "nature treasures." Fallen leaves, speckled stones, tiny pinecones, acorns, flower petals, stray feathers. When we get home, she'll dump everything out on the porch and sort it into piles. Sometimes she builds fairy houses. Sometimes it becomes a crown. Sometimes she just studies everything in silence, like she's deciphering the language of the woods. Whatever her imagination dreams up, it begins with wonder.

And that's exactly what I want for her.

In a world moving faster by the day, where children are often scheduled from sunup to sundown and faced with too many screens, the chance to be still, to explore, to notice—that's a gift. These unstructured outdoor hours aren't a break from learning. They are learning. They offer something that worksheets and digital flashcards can't: presence, freedom, and connection.

It's not just about nature. It's about what happens in nature. Children learn their boundaries when we don't define every inch of the play. They discover what their bodies are capable of when we stop narrating every move. They take risks and fall sometimes. They scrape knees. They test how far they can climb, how fast they can run. And in doing so, they become more aware of themselves, of others, of the earth beneath them.

And it's not just Lucy.

I've watched the same wonder reshape Anderson, too. On weekends when he stays with us and has time away from screens, something amazing happens. His entire demeanor softens. He goes from quiet and withdrawn to chatty and hilarious. He becomes more present, more connected, more himself. Unplugging doesn't just clear his mind—it revives his spirit. It's amazing what God's world can do for the soul.

He and Lucy will play outside for hours—racing each other through the yard with the dogs bounding behind them, inventing games, or tossing the football back and forth. Anderson teaches Lucy the names of players and teams and walks her through game strategies with all the enthusiasm of a future coach. And when they finally tumble back indoors, they're sweaty, out of breath, and full of smiles—the good kind, the kind born from movement and shared joy.

Not every moment is picturesque. Play, especially outdoor play, has a wild side. And that's a good thing.

We've tried to give Anderson and Lucy room to experience that—to learn how to handle conflict, how to share leadership in a game, how to take a deep breath when they don't get their way. These moments, especially with peers, are full of teachable tension. They're the kind of moments where parents often feel tempted to step in. But when the risks are low and the stakes are social, I've found that holding back often teaches the most. Letting kids experience the discomfort of disagreement or the joy of reconciliation is essential. These are the roots of emotional intelligence.

Nature has also offered a more subtle kind of wisdom: the understanding of seasons.

Lucy has noticed that some trees lose their leaves while others stay green. She's pointed out how caterpillars disappear only to reappear later, transformed. She sees the way summer brings butterflies and winter brings stillness. And we talk about it—not just as science, but as something sacred.

I remind her that life works the same way.

There are seasons of growth and seasons of rest. Times when we feel full of energy and times when everything feels gray. But just like spring always follows winter, joy always returns. This rhythm, built into the world by the same God who made her, teaches her to sit with sadness when it comes and to trust that it won't last forever. That her feelings are real, but not permanent. That light always comes again.

These days in nature, these long afternoons of play, they aren't just for passing time. They're shaping Lucy's heart—and Anderson's too. They're helping them grow in empathy, awareness, patience, and strength. They're giving them memories made of sun-warmed skin, muddy shoes, and wind in their hair. They're giving them time to become.

The truth is, we all need more of this.

More wild moments. More space to breathe. More time to listen to the birds and follow the butterflies and look up at the clouds and say, "Look what God made today." Because the wild is not just where we wander, it's where we remember who we are.

The beauty of learning in the wild is that there's no timeline—just curiosity, wonder, and growth at the child's pace. And that's a lesson I've carried into every corner of our educational life. Because once you let go of the pressure to "keep up," you begin to see learning for what it truly is: not a race to the next milestone, but a path toward deep understanding. That's what the next chapter is all about—letting go of checklists and choosing mastery instead.

Reflections Pages

1. A moment from this chapter that stood out to me:

2. How this moment connects to my own story, family, or childhood:

3. A belief, habit, or pattern I noticed in myself:

4. A more compassionate or truthful way of seeing this part of my story is:

5. One practical step I want to take this week is:

6. What might get in the way:

7. How I can support myself when it feels hard:

8. A Bible verse this chapter reminds me of and why:

____

____

____

9. A prayer, affirmation, or intention I want to carry forward:

____

____

____

Take what serves you, release what doesn't. Healing and learning are slow, holy work — and you are doing beautifully.

Chapter 13

Mastery, Not Milestones

"Do not conform to the pattern of this world, but be transformed by the renewing of your mind."

—Romans 12:2

In traditional education, everything is measured by milestones. What should a child know by age six? By grade three? What percentage did they get on the test? Are they "on track"? But when you step outside that framework—even just slightly—you begin to realize how arbitrary those markers really are.

Children are not machines. They don't develop on conveyor belts. Some will read at four, others at eight, and both are equally capable of becoming lifelong learners. The goal isn't to check every box at the right time. The goal is understanding, confidence, and joy. Mastery over milestones.

This truth has been clear in our home, where two children—raised with similar values and deep love—learn in radically different ways. Lucy picks up concepts quickly. Learning lights her up. She remembers what she reads and often connects dots before I can even ask the question. Anderson, on the other hand, has to work harder. Like me, learning hasn't always come easily for him. He has to dig deeper, push through more resistance, and stretch himself in ways that aren't always visible on a worksheet. But here's the thing: the effort is the achievement.

It's been such a reminder that kids are not meant to be compared. They're meant to be known.

Anderson has taught me that mastery isn't always measured by ease or speed. Sometimes it's measured by persistence. By the way, a child keeps going even when the path feels uphill. And because his journey has been harder, his victories feel especially meaningful. He may not always meet traditional timelines, but when he gets something—when it clicks—you can see the pride light up his whole face. He's not just checking a box. He's owning the learning.

It's also why we've been intentional in shaping his educational environment. When we noticed he was being pushed along in school without true understanding, we—together with his mom—found a mastery-based charter school where 80% is the standard to move forward. Not to add pressure, but to ensure that every step forward is on solid ground. Anderson thrives when the focus is on depth, not deadlines. And though his progress may be slower than Lucy's, it is no less valuable.

Kids learn differently — humans learn differently — and honoring that truth has shaped everything about how we teach both Lucy and Anderson. Lucy learns best when lessons are rich with story, connection, and imagery. Give her a narrative, and she lights up. Anderson, on the other hand, needs clarity and structure. Too many layers can overwhelm him, but when the steps are clear and the expectations grounded, he thrives. Their strengths aren't identical, but they're equally worthy. Mastery isn't about learning the same way — it's about learning in your way.

That's the beauty of knowing your learners. They are not the same—and they shouldn't be taught the same way. Anderson doesn't need the story to make a lesson meaningful. He needs the tools to feel successful, confident, and grounded in what he's learning. And when he has that—when the path is clear, and the expectations are reasonable—he rises to it. He shines in his own right.

So yes—Lucy has hit milestone after milestone "ahead of schedule"—but not because she's some kind of prodigy. She's not. She's a bright, curious, deeply loved child whose mom simply watches, listens, and responds. I don't force her to do things she's not ready for—but I also don't lower the bar just to make things easier. I set it just high enough for her to stretch, and I let her know I believe she can reach it. That belief—hers and mine—makes all the difference.

I remind both kids often: understanding matters more than speed. We don't rush through a lesson to stay "on grade level." If a concept doesn't click right away, we pause, review, and try a new approach. Not to delay progress, but to deepen roots. Learning isn't about ticking boxes—it's about truly knowing something. And when you know it, no one can take it from you.

Mastery builds confidence. Not the kind that puffs up, but the kind that anchors. And when either of them finds something challenging, we don't see it as a failure or a reason to stop. We adjust. We slow down. We get creative. But we keep going. Because real learning isn't about finishing fast—it's about finishing well.

And honestly, this mindset has shaped me, too. It's helped me release the pressure of comparison—the temptation to measure Lucy or Anderson against someone else's timeline. They are not on anyone else's journey. They are on theirs. And my job isn't to push them ahead or hold them back. It's to walk beside them, celebrate their progress, and remind them that mastery is worth the time it takes.

So we learn at their pace. We dive deep. We chase rabbit trails. And sometimes, we stay on a lesson longer than the guide suggests—not because they're behind, but because there's more to explore.

It's not always clean or easy. Some days, it's messy and slow and full of doubt. But I've come to believe that's where the magic happens. In the space between what's expected and what's real—in the light that reflects when a child truly gets something, not because a test says so, but because they've lived it, practiced it, owned it.

That's mastery. And that's the kind of education I'll choose—every time.

Reflections Pages

1. A moment from this chapter that stood out to me:

2. How this moment connects to my own story, family, or childhood:

3. A belief, habit, or pattern I noticed in myself:

4. A more compassionate or truthful way of seeing this part of my story is:

5. One practical step I want to take this week is:

6. What might get in the way:

7. How I can support myself when it feels hard:

8. A Bible verse this chapter reminds me of and why:

____

____

____

9. A prayer, affirmation, or intention I want to carry forward:

____

____

____

Take what serves you, release what doesn't. Healing and learning are slow, holy work — and you are doing beautifully.

Chapter 14

Sacred Slowness

"In repentance and rest is your salvation, in quietness and trust is your strength."

—Isaiah 30:15

Choosing mastery meant choosing a slower pace—one that gave space for curiosity, rest, and the sacred way of life that comes from simply being together.

There's a rhythm to childhood that's easy to miss when life moves too fast. It doesn't sound like a school bell or feel like a countdown to bedtime. It's gentler than that. Quieter. It sounds like belly laughs over breakfast. It feels like holding hands during a walk with nowhere to be. It shows up in the pauses—the white space around the moments that matter most.

I didn't always know how to protect that space. Before I became a mother, my life was packed with jobs, deadlines, calendars, and obligations. Productivity was the measure of a "good day." Rest felt like something you earned once everything was done. But motherhood shifted all of that. And homeschooling deepened it.

It's not that we don't have a schedule. We do. But we're no longer slaves to it. If Lucy's curiosity sparks a rabbit trail, we follow it. If she's having a rough morning, we adjust. If the weather is perfect, we take school outside—or ditch the books for a nature walk and call it science. This flexibility isn't laziness. It's intentionality. It's choosing presence over pressure.

I get to witness the milestones—not just hear about them secondhand. I'm there when a tricky concept finally clicks. I'm there for the impromptu dance performances in the living room, the stories she writes unprompted, the questions she asks that take us deep into topics I never expected. I don't have to ask how her day went. I'm in it with her.

And that—more than any curriculum or checklist—is the radical gift of time. Time to listen. Time to rest. Time to let a moment stretch, instead of rushing it along.

There's so much messaging in our culture about hustling, optimizing, and achieving. Even childhood isn't immune. Enrichment classes, sports, academic benchmarks—it's easy to feel like you're always running to keep up. But children aren't meant to be hurried. They're meant to unfold.

When we slow down, we notice more. We connect more. We savor more. And we create space for God to work—not in the frantic noise, but in the stillness.

Of course, there are still busy days. Appointments, errands, places to be. But those aren't the norm—they're the exception. Our norm is margin. Our default is peace.

That doesn't mean we always feel peaceful. We still have hard days, cranky mornings, and emotional meltdowns (sometimes hers, sometimes mine). But we've learned how to return to calm. To take deep breaths. To go outside. To read aloud on the couch when everything else feels like too much. We've learned how to rest with each other.

And I think that's what sacred slowness really is. It's not about doing less—it's about doing what matters, with intention and grace. It's about making room for the kind of growth that can't be rushed.

One day, Lucy will grow up. The pace of our days will shift again. But I hope she carries this with her—that slowing down isn't weakness. It's wisdom. That rest isn't laziness. It's fuel. And that life isn't a race. It's a walk with purpose.

And if she ever forgets, I hope the memory of these long mornings and unhurried afternoons will whisper it back to her:

You were never meant to be hurried, my love. You were made to bloom in your own time.

So we choose to slow down, not just for the sake of rest, but to make room for the kind of deep, dignified growth that can't be rushed.

Reflections Pages

1. A moment from this chapter that stood out to me:

2. How this moment connects to my own story, family, or childhood:

3. A belief, habit, or pattern I noticed in myself:

4. A more compassionate or truthful way of seeing this part of my story is:

5. One practical step I want to take this week is:

6. What might get in the way:

7. How I can support myself when it feels hard:

8. A Bible verse this chapter reminds me of and why:

____

____

____

9. A prayer, affirmation, or intention I want to carry forward:

____

____

____

Take what serves you, release what doesn't. Healing and learning are slow, holy work — and you are doing beautifully.

Chapter 15
Not My Shining Moment

"But he said to me, 'My grace is sufficient for you, for my power is made perfect in weakness.'Therefore I will boast all the more gladly about my weaknesses, so that Christ's power may rest on me."

—2 Corinthians 12:9

I wish I could say I've always parented with calm composure and Christ-like grace.

But then there was the day I jumped up and down like a wild woman, arms flailing, yelling at my daughter at the top of my lungs. Spoiler alert: not my shining moment.

Lucy had always been easygoing when it came to babysitters, grandparents, and even her extracurriculars. She never clung to me. Never cried at drop-off. Never fussed if I ran inside quickly to grab something I'd forgotten—her water bottle, a snack, or occasionally my sanity—while she waited in the car. But one Saturday morning, that all changed. Richard and Lucy were heading out for their usual grocery-store tradition when he realized he'd left something in the house. He ran in to grab it—and got momentarily sidetracked by a quick question from Anderson. The whole thing took less than a few minutes. But to Lucy, it felt like forever. When Richard returned to the car, she was sobbing.

He comforted her and thought it was a one-time thing. But in the days that followed, something shifted. Lucy suddenly began panicking any time I walked away. When I had to run back into the house to grab her water bottle, she cried. At her usual activity drop-off, where she had always been fine, she clung to me. Soon, it wasn't just drop-offs. It was being on a different level of the house! She needed constant reassurance that I wasn't going to leave her.

I tried everything—talking, comforting, explaining, praying. I told her God was always with her. I reminded her of the thousands of times I had kept my promises. But nothing worked. It only escalated. I felt helpless. I even considered calling a child psychologist. And somewhere in all of it, I started to unravel.

Then came that day.

Lucy was sitting at the table, working on her schoolwork. I told her I needed to quickly let the dogs out in the backyard. "Stay here," I said gently. "You've got this. I'll be right back."

She nodded.

Seconds later, I glanced up and saw her peeking through the basement window, having quietly snuck down after me. I stepped inside and watched her bolt back upstairs. I hollered up the steps, exasperated: "Lucy, you have to listen and stay up there! I'm only in the backyard!"

I turned toward the door again—and heard her tiny feet racing across the floor, headed back down. That's when I snapped. I pretended to step outside, and as she came flying down the stairs, I met her with all the chaos that had been building up inside me.

I lost it.

I jumped up and down like an unhinged kangaroo, flailing my arms and shouting, "Why won't you just LISTEN to me?! Get upstairs NOW!"

Lucy ran upstairs, no doubt in shock over my horrific behavior—and I just stood there, stunned.

The moment it was over, the shame poured in. I had let my emotions take the wheel. I wasn't in control—I was exhausted and overwhelmed. And instead of helping Lucy regain her confidence, I had just confirmed her fear. I sat there, stunned by my own outburst. As the rage drained, the guilt took root.

Was she going to be scarred for life? Would she ever feel safe again? Had I just undone years of intentional parenting with a single tantrum of my own?

Eventually, I dragged myself upstairs. I told Lucy I needed ten minutes to gather myself and that we'd talk afterward. When I came back, I sat across from her at the table and took a deep breath.

"Lucy," I said, "there's no excuse for how I acted earlier. It doesn't matter what happened or what you did or didn't do—I should never speak to you that way. I lost control. I'm really sorry. You don't have to forgive me today or even tomorrow, but I hope you'll be able to forgive me someday."

I told her I wasn't perfect (clearly). That I was trying to help her feel safe again, but I was also having a hard time. I poured my heart out, hoping it would land softly.

She looked at me with a little smile and said, "Mom, it's totally ok… but did you know you could JUMP that high?!"

I blinked.

Then I laughed.

Then we laughed.

And in that laughter, I felt something crack open—something holy.

"Wait… is that seriously all you saw in that wild moment?" I asked, half-laughing, half-weeping. "You didn't see a mom monster? You just saw how high I could JUMP?"

That was the moment God's grace broke through. Not with a lecture or a lesson, but with a little girl's wide-eyed wonder—somehow able to see past my failure and find something funny. She didn't see rage. She saw me. The real me. The one she knew deep down. And through her eyes, I saw it too.

It wasn't the blessing I deserved—but it was exactly the one my heart needed—a daughter who forgave without being asked. Who knew me so well, she could tune out the parts that weren't really me… and find something beautiful hiding inside the mess.

It wasn't my shining moment.

But it became a sacred one.

Because Lucy didn't see a mom who was flawless—she saw a mom who was honest. A mom who lost her temper and then came back to own it. A mom who said sorry. And apparently, a mom who could jump!

And maybe that's what she needed most.

Reflections Pages

1. A moment from this chapter that stood out to me:

2. How this moment connects to my own story, family, or childhood:

3. A belief, habit, or pattern I noticed in myself:

4. A more compassionate or truthful way of seeing this part of my story is:

____

____

____

____

5. One practical step I want to take this week is:

____

____

____

6. What might get in the way:

____

____

____

7. How I can support myself when it feels hard:

____

____

____

8. A Bible verse this chapter reminds me of and why:

____

____

____

9. A prayer, affirmation, or intention I want to carry forward:

____

____

____

Take what serves you, release what doesn't. Healing and learning are slow, holy work — and you are doing beautifully.

Chapter 16

Rooted and Respected

Discipline with Dignity

"No discipline seems pleasant at the time, but painful. Later on, however, it produces a harvest of righteousness and peace for those who have been trained by it."

–Hebrews 12:11

There's a common misconception that discipline means domination—that to be "in charge," a parent must raise their voice, lose their cool, or demand obedience through fear. But I've learned, through years of training dogs, teaching children, and raising my own, that true discipline has nothing to do with fear. Real leadership is calm, clear, and consistent. And it begins with dignity.

As a dog trainer, I learned early on that behavior is communication. A dog who jumps, growls, or disobeys isn't "bad"—they're either confused, overstimulated, or lacking structure. And the solution is not to get louder or harsher. It's to get clearer. To be calm, assertive, and in tune with what the animal needs. That lesson stayed with me when I stepped into a classroom as a teacher, and again when I stepped into motherhood.

Notice I said "assertive" clarity. That absolutely does not mean being a pushover—and it certainly doesn't mean adopting the trendy model of "gentle parenting," which I wholeheartedly disagree with. One of the most powerful principles I've carried with me is the importance of matching intensity. If your child is operating at a level 7—emotionally charged, angry, or spiraling—and you respond at a level 4, they can't hear you. They won't respect you. Your voice won't register. On the other hand, if you come in hot at a level 10, overwhelming them with anger, you might get obedience—but it will come from fear, not understanding. Neither extreme leads to long-term trust or growth.

The goal is to meet them at their level with a calm, firm energy—assertive, never aggressive. Stay at that level until they de-escalate. Once they've come down, that's when the real work begins. Now, you can speak to them with tenderness, guide them with reason, and offer consequences that make sense. This isn't about punishment—it's about preparation. Helping them become people of character who know how to self-regulate.

One evening, Lucy had a rough moment while we were out to dinner with friends. She was hungry and impatient, and it showed. She was making faces, sighing loudly, and fidgeting with everything on the table. She loves a show called Jane, inspired by the life and work of Jane Goodall, and I had told her earlier that if she had a good evening, she could watch an episode after dinner.

As her behavior started to spiral, I leaned in close—discreetly, so I could preserve her dignity—and said calmly but firmly, "Keep this up, and there will be no Jane tonight." The warning worked… for about five minutes. Then the whining and impatience crept back in.

I leaned in again. "You just chose to lose the privilege of watching Jane. Continue, and we'll be leaving the table. You'll sit in the car with me while Dad finishes his meal."

Everything about me in that moment—my tone, my posture, my eye contact—communicated that I meant what I said. I didn't need to raise my voice. I didn't need to lecture. I just needed to be clear and follow through. She knew I would.

She didn't get to watch Jane that night. That was a natural consequence. But she did collect herself and was able to enjoy dinner politely with us—because she made that choice. That's the point I always try to circle back to: she is in control of her emotions. And with that truth comes responsibility, but also empowerment.

She did ask if she could still watch Jane because she had turned things around at dinner. And while I praised her for her change in behavior, I held firm. I reminded her that she had lost the Jane privilege, but because she chose to reset and show self-control, she got to enjoy something else that is a privilege: a nice family dinner. It's so tempting in those moments to backtrack, to let the consequence slide because they've recovered. But when we do that, we teach them that our words don't really matter—and next time, they won't believe we mean what we say.

But discipline isn't just about catching the wrong behavior—it's also about catching the right. It's easy to spot and call out the missteps, but if we're not careful, we miss the quiet moments when our children are doing exactly what they should. Those are the moments that deserve our full attention. When we notice and praise the good—the kindness, the patience, the effort—they light up. That smile, that small burst of pride, isn't just heart-melting—it's powerful. Because in that moment, they're being seen for their goodness. And when a child is acknowledged for doing right, they are far more likely to repeat it. It meets the same desire for attention that often fuels misbehavior, but in a life-giving, character-building way.

It's one of the greatest lessons we can give our children: the ability to regulate their emotional state. There's not much in this life we can control—but our attitude, our self-discipline, our response to difficulty? That's within our reach.

But it's not easy. Mastering your emotions is like building any other skill. You want to be better at basketball? You practice. Want to become a better cook? You'll go through messes, mistakes, and a mountain of dirty dishes before you start to get it right. Emotional regulation is no different—it's a muscle, and it must be worked regularly.

It takes practice. It takes grit. It takes grace.

And it starts with us—the parents, the leaders, the ones who teach by example. We don't just talk about self-control. We show it. We pause before we react. We breathe before we correct. We separate the child from the behavior, and we lead with love.

In our home, discipline is not about asserting power. It's about establishing trust. Our children are not projects to fix—they're people to guide. And when correction comes with dignity, consistency, and compassion, they don't just learn how to behave. They learn how to belong.

And that, I believe, is the heart of it all.

That same intentionality—meeting our children with calm consistency, giving them space to grow—also shaped the choices we made about how our home would feel. It wasn't just about how we handled conflict. It was about what filled their eyes, what captured their attention, and how we carved out space for connection and imagination.

One of the most powerful ways we've done that? We put screens in their proper place—minimized, not glorified—so that real life could take center stage.

Reflections Pages

1. A moment from this chapter that stood out to me:

2. How this moment connects to my own story, family, or childhood:

3. A belief, habit, or pattern I noticed in myself:

4. A more compassionate or truthful way of seeing this part of my story is:

5. One practical step I want to take this week is:

6. What might get in the way:

7. How I can support myself when it feels hard:

8. A Bible verse this chapter reminds me of and why:

____

____

____

9. A prayer, affirmation, or intention I want to carry forward:

____

____

____

Take what serves you, release what doesn't. Healing and learning are slow, holy work — and you are doing beautifully.

Part 4: Choosing Light in a Complicated World

In a culture that moves fast and shouts loud, this part is about choosing a different way—one rooted in connection, intention, and peace. It's about the rhythms of family life that nourish instead of drain, the countercultural decisions that raise eyebrows, and the sacred gift of tuning out noise to tune into each other.

In this section, I'll share the intentional rhythms and countercultural choices we've made—from minimizing screens to resisting pressure, from nurturing health to rewriting the script of our own childhoods—all in pursuit of raising children who are rooted, whole, and free to shine.

Chapter 17

Minimal Screens, Maximum Connection

"Everything is permissible for me—but not everything is beneficial."

—1 Corinthians 10:23

In our home, screens are not the enemy—but they're not in charge, either.

From the very beginning, Richard and I were intentional about how we introduced technology to our kids. When Lucy was a baby, I was pretty emphatic: no screens. For the first two years of her life, the only light she stared at came from a sunbeam through the window or the flicker of candlelight at dinner. I knew the science. I knew the stats. But more than that, I knew how precious these early years were—and I didn't want her eyes on a screen when they could be on the world instead.

After she turned two, we began easing in gently. A National Geographic show here and there—a quiet thirty minutes a couple of times a week. When she was about two and a half, I introduced Daniel Tiger. I liked the values it taught. It was calm. Slow.

Thoughtful. The screen didn't change scenes every 0.3 seconds or shout in neon chaos. It felt like a gentle invitation into the digital world—not an onslaught.

But even now, Lucy doesn't use screens in the car. Not for errands. Not for school pickup lines. Not at restaurants, grocery stores, or doctors' offices. Screens aren't our solution for waiting, fidgeting, or quieting discomfort. And I know that's not always the easiest path—but it's the one we've chosen.

Why? Because I believe boredom is a skill. And like any skill, it needs to be practiced.

When kids are constantly given something to watch or swipe or scroll, they don't learn what to do with stillness. They miss the muscle-building moments of having to entertain themselves, to sit with their thoughts, to create something out of nothing. That quiet restlessness? That's where imagination lives. That's where self-control grows. That's where real connection takes root.

Screens train the brain to expect novelty—every fraction of a second, a new image, a new sound, a new thrill. But the real world doesn't work like that. The real world is slower. It's quieter. It requires something of you. So what happens when a child grows up immersed in a hyper-stimulated digital environment and is then asked to sit in a classroom and pay attention for an hour? Or have a real conversation with someone face-to-face? Or simply sit in their own company without distraction? That's not just difficult—it can feel impossible.

We've seen the difference firsthand.

On the weekends, when Anderson is with us, we keep screens to a minimum. And something beautiful happens. He shifts. At first, it's subtle—but then, like watching a seed sprout after rain, the change becomes clear. He becomes more talkative. More playful. More connected. We do puzzles together. We build Legos. We play board games, read books aloud, cook meals, and yes—sometimes we're bored.

But boredom, too, is a gift.

Anderson starts telling jokes. Lucy starts building obstacle courses out of couch cushions. They race with the dogs in the backyard. They grab a book for the car. He teaches her all about football stats and game strategies while she shows him how to make pinecone tea for the imaginary forest creatures they've discovered. They're sweaty, out of breath, and full of smiles. Their cheeks are pink. Their hearts are light. And not a screen in sight.

These moments remind me that connection isn't found in convenience—it's found in the messy, unplugged spaces between tasks and timelines. In shared laughter, in eye contact, in a puzzle piece that finally fits.

I'm not against technology. It's a tool—and a powerful one. But in our home, it's not the foundation of our childhood memories. That honor belongs to backyard adventures, books, flour-dusted countertops, late-night stories, and board games that last too long. It belongs to curiosity, presence, and the deep, quiet joy of being fully here.

Because when we minimize screens, we make space for something greater.

We make space for connection. For creativity. For the kind of family life that doesn't need to be charged at night—just cherished.

And as we've found rhythm in these unplugged moments—shaped by boredom, creativity, and connection—we've also discovered how vital our daily rhythms are overall. What we eat, how we move, how we spend our mornings and evenings… it all matters. In the next chapter, we'll look at how food, focus, and family rhythms play a role in shaping not just a child's health, but their sense of belonging and stability, too.

Because what we do every day isn't just a habit—it's a legacy.

Let's build one worth passing down—one bite, one breath, one quiet rhythm at a time.

Reflections Pages

1. A moment from this chapter that stood out to me:

2. How this moment connects to my own story, family, or childhood:

3. A belief, habit, or pattern I noticed in myself:

4. A more compassionate or truthful way of seeing this part of my story is:

____

____

____

____

5. One practical step I want to take this week is:

____

____

____

6. What might get in the way:

____

____

____

7. How I can support myself when it feels hard:

____

____

____

8. A Bible verse this chapter reminds me of and why:

____

____

____

9. A prayer, affirmation, or intention I want to carry forward:

____

____

____

Take what serves you, release what doesn't. Healing and learning are slow, holy work — and you are doing beautifully.

Chapter 18

Food, Focus, and Family Rhythms

Nurturing the Whole Child

"Or do you not know that your body is a temple of the Holy Spirit within you…? Therefore glorify God in your body."

—1 Corinthians 6:19–20

In our home, nourishment isn't just about eating—it's about equipping. Food fuels focus. Routines shape peace. And daily rhythms ground our family in ways that nourish the body, mind, and spirit. Just as we are intentional about how we educate our children, we're just as intentional about how we feed them—and ourselves.

Every morning, before the hustle of the day begins, Richard and I work out together. It's our time to sweat, connect, and set the tone. It's not just about physical fitness—it's about being the kind of parents who model discipline, health, and vitality. Our kids see that. They see us choosing movement. They see us choosing real food. They see that health isn't something you do when it's convenient—it's a lifestyle you build, brick by brick.

We don't subscribe to restrictive diets. We honor all the macronutrients—carbohydrates, proteins, and fats—as essential gifts that serve different purposes in the body. Carbs fuel the brain and muscles, aid digestion, and deliver nutrients. Protein helps build and preserve muscle, supports bone and skin health. And fats—good fats like olive oil, butter, and avocado—support heart health, brain function, and help us absorb vital vitamins. We don't fear food. We understand it. And we teach that to our children from a place of respect, not restriction.

That means no processed sugar as a norm, though we do embrace natural sugars in moderation—honey, maple syrup, fresh fruit. Lucy had her first candy bar at four years old (and I cringed the entire time). To this day, she usually doesn't enjoy the taste of overly processed sweets. Once, after a dance class, the teacher handed out lollipops. Lucy politely asked, "This isn't good for me. Can I have a sticker instead?" Her teacher was floored—and I was quietly proud, not because of the choice itself, but because of the why behind it. She understood how food made her feel. She was learning to listen to her body.

It's not about never indulging. We love food in this house—deeply. But we want it to taste good, not just to the tongue, but to the whole body. And we talk about that, especially when Lucy does have something processed. You can practically watch the shift. Her calm demeanor gives way to restlessness. She struggles to regulate her body and her emotions. I ask her how she feels, and she's learning to recognize the connection: "My body feels crazy," she once said after eating a birthday cupcake. That awareness? That's the goal. Not fear. Not shame. Just understanding.

We've also chosen to avoid fast food as a rule. As I write this, Lucy is just shy of six years old and has never eaten from McDonald's or Burger King. The only "fast food" we eat comes from places that serve real, unprocessed meals. Food made by people, not machines. Food that doesn't require a decoder ring to understand the ingredients list.

This rhythm of respect—for food, for feelings, for focus—carries over into everything we do. And it's not just Lucy who benefits from it.

On the weekends, when Anderson is with us, we carry these rhythms into our time together. He genuinely enjoys helping in the kitchen—whether he's flipping pancakes on a Saturday morning or seasoning the chicken for dinner. Cooking becomes a shared experience, a chance to talk, laugh, and teach. Just like with Lucy, we invite him to pay attention to how food makes him feel, helping him connect nourishment with energy, mood, and well-being.

It's not about perfection. There are weekends with s'mores by the fire, pizza nights, and plenty of silly snacks. But even those moments are rooted in togetherness. The treat isn't just the food—it's the atmosphere. We play board games. We linger at the table. We let conversations wander from silly to serious. The food matters, but it's the connection we crave most. The treat isn't just on the plate—it's in the presence.

Because in the end, the table isn't just where we eat. It's where we talk, laugh, and belong. It's where conversations flow as freely as the ingredients, and where simple meals become sacred memories.

Our family rhythms may not look like everyone else's. But they are life-giving. They are grounding. And they are intentional. Because raising healthy, whole, vibrant kids means nurturing more than just the mind, it means nourishing the soul.

We've built a home rooted in intention—but the moment we share that light beyond our walls, we're reminded that not everyone will receive it with kindness. And yet, that doesn't mean we stop shining.

Reflections Pages

1. A moment from this chapter that stood out to me:

2. How this moment connects to my own story, family, or childhood:

3. A belief, habit, or pattern I noticed in myself:

4. A more compassionate or truthful way of seeing this part of my story is:

____

____

____

____

5. One practical step I want to take this week is:

____

____

____

6. What might get in the way:

____

____

____

7. How I can support myself when it feels hard:

____

____

____

8. A Bible verse this chapter reminds me of and why:

____

____

____

9. A prayer, affirmation, or intention I want to carry forward:

____

____

____

Take what serves you, release what doesn't. Healing and learning are slow, holy work — and you are doing beautifully.

Chapter 19

When the World Pushes Back

On Criticism, Comparison, and Choosing Grace Anyway

"Am I now trying to win the approval of human beings, or of God? Or am I trying to please people? If I were still trying to please people, I would not be a servant of Christ."

—Galatians 1:10

There's a quiet kind of courage required to live differently. And an even louder kind needed to share about it publicly.

I remember the morning I posted the photo of Lucy starting third grade. She sat tall on the table we use for homeschooling in her favorite dress, beaming with excitement. She was five years old and already flourishing in a curriculum designed for kids several years older—not because we were racing ahead, but because we had followed her natural pace. I shared the moment in a homeschooling group filled with other Christian moms using the same curriculum, thinking it might spark hope or encouragement.

Wow, was I ever in for a surprise!

Roughly eighty percent of the comments were kind. Encouraging. Celebratory. But then came the other twenty percent that knocked the wind out of me.

One woman suggested my daughter had a rare disease—one with a 15-year life expectancy—and that's why she appeared "different." Another accused me of being intentionally cruel, suggesting my post was meant to hurt moms whose children weren't as "advanced." Some insisted Lucy was "obviously gifted," and therefore shouldn't be compared to "normal" kids. One even said I was being insensitive to the parents of children with learning disabilities.

That's when I stepped in.

I thanked the women who understood the heart behind the post—a mom proud of her daughter, a mom offering hope to others wondering if homeschool could really work. A mom simply sharing a light.

And then, with equal clarity, I responded to the rest.

I explained that not only do I have a learning disability myself, but so does my beautiful son—my bonus boy, Anderson. He has cerebral palsy and a chromosome deletion. Learning is incredibly hard for him. Retaining information is exhausting. And yet, he's one of the most joyful, steady-hearted people I know.

He has never felt overshadowed by Lucy's light. Not once. Why? Because in our home, academic achievement is just one way to shine—not the only way. We praise effort. We praise empathy. We praise character, grit, self-control, and the courage it takes to keep going when something doesn't come easily. We praise Anderson's talent for sports—his incredible ability to throw a football with pinpoint accuracy. Lucy couldn't compete with that if she tried, and she knows it. So she cheers him on. And when we praise him for that gift, we remind him to thank God for it—just like we remind Lucy to thank God for her quick comprehension and love of learning.

We've worked hard to cultivate a home where comparison has no fertile soil. Each child is celebrated for who they are—not who they aren't. And when someone else's light shines brightly, we don't squint or shield our eyes. We say, "Look at what God is doing."

After I said my piece, I quietly left the group.

Because I don't need that kind of negativity in my life, I don't need people who twist celebration into condemnation. I don't need to justify my joy or sanitize my story to make it more palatable for others. I can share from a place of gratitude and confidence, knowing that God sees the heart—and He is the only one I'm living to please.

And maybe that's the hardest part of homeschooling, or parenting differently in general: not the long days or curriculum choices, but the courage it takes to stand firm when the world pushes back, when strangers misunderstand you, when friends or even family question your path. When people say things that are cruel or careless or just plain wrong.

But here's what I've learned:

When the world pushes back, you don't have to push harder. You don't have to convince them. You don't even have to stay in the conversation. You just have to root yourself in truth—and stay there.

Lucy doesn't owe the world a slower pace just to make others comfortable. Anderson doesn't owe the world easier milestones to prove his worth. And I don't owe the world a watered-down version of what works in our home.

We are not raising our children to be palatable. We are raising them to be purposeful. And that means their paths will look different—and that difference might provoke discomfort. But that's okay.

Because when the world pushes back, we don't shrink—we rise. Not in defiance, but with quiet determination to live differently. To raise differently. To learn differently. In the next chapter, I'll share how that quiet rebellion took root in our home—where we began rewriting not only the world's expectations, but the generational stories that had shaped us.

Reflections Pages

1. A moment from this chapter that stood out to me:

2. How this moment connects to my own story, family, or childhood:

3. A belief, habit, or pattern I noticed in myself:

4. A more compassionate or truthful way of seeing this part of my story is:

5. One practical step I want to take this week is:

6. What might get in the way:

7. How I can support myself when it feels hard:

8. A Bible verse this chapter reminds me of and why:

____

____

____

9. A prayer, affirmation, or intention I want to carry forward:

____

____

____

Take what serves you, release what doesn't. Healing and learning are slow, holy work — and you are doing beautifully.

Chapter 20

Rewriting the Script

"Do not conform to the pattern of this world, but be transformed by the renewing of your mind."

—Romans 12:2

There comes a moment in every parent's journey where you're faced with a choice: repeat what you know, or rewrite what you've lived. For me, that choice showed up early. I knew I wanted something different for my children—something more life-giving than the patterns I grew up with.

Growing up, school wasn't joyful. It was pressure. It was a shame. It was always feeling like I was behind, even when I was trying my hardest. It took years for me to realize that my struggle wasn't a lack of intelligence—it was a lack of understanding in the system around me. And while I eventually found my voice, my confidence, and even my brilliance, I had to fight for it.

I don't want my children to have to fight to be seen.

Homeschooling gave me the opportunity to rewrite the script—not just for Lucy and Anderson, but for myself. It let me lean into curiosity instead of comparison, depth instead of deadlines. In our home, learning isn't something to survive. It's something to savor.

That doesn't mean we never face challenges. Of course we do. But challenges aren't treated like personal failures. They're treated as part of the process. We slow down. We reassess. We try again. And we speak grace over every effort.

Rewriting the script means praising effort over outcome. It means celebrating when something is hard—and they don't quit. It means pulling away from the pressure to perform and instead teaching our children to learn for the joy of understanding.

It also means addressing the stories we've internalized. The "I'm not smart enough," or "I'll never get this," or "I'm just bad at math." We don't let those narratives go unchecked. We talk about them. We reframe them. We help our children speak truth over themselves.

And we model it, too.

Because healing doesn't just happen in our kids, it happens in us, as we choose something different. As we trade the anxiety of perfectionism for the peace of progress. As we remember that worth has never depended on performance, and it never will.

This chapter of our life isn't just about teaching differently. It's about living differently. It's about making sure our children know that they are more than a test score, more than a behavior chart, more than a grade.

They are fully known, fully loved, and free to learn at their own pace—with joy.

Because when we change the script, we don't just rewrite the story for one child—we set a new tone for generations to come. We become the kind of family where identity is rooted in truth, where mistakes are part of learning, and where light doesn't flicker under pressure—it shines brighter.

And that light? It doesn't just glow in the moments of academic growth—it shines most in the daily rhythms of home, where presence becomes the greatest teacher of all.

Reflections Pages

1. A moment from this chapter that stood out to me:

2. How this moment connects to my own story, family, or childhood:

3. A belief, habit, or pattern I noticed in myself:

4. A more compassionate or truthful way of seeing this part of my story is:

____

____

____

____

5. One practical step I want to take this week is:

____

____

____

6. What might get in the way:

____

____

____

7. How I can support myself when it feels hard:

____

____

____

8. A Bible verse this chapter reminds me of and why:

---

9. A prayer, affirmation, or intention I want to carry forward:

Take what serves you, release what doesn't. Healing and learning are slow, holy work — and you are doing beautifully.

Chapter 21

The Role of the Parent as Teacher

The best curriculum in the world can't outshine the power of a present, purposeful parent.

"Start children off on the way they should go, and even when they are old they will not turn from it."

—Proverbs 22:6

In our home, homeschooling isn't just something we try to squeeze in around errands and activities—it's the anchor of our daily rhythm. We don't homeschool when it's convenient; we build the rest of our day around it. That structure brings a beautiful sense of peace and purpose to our mornings. We start with snuggles, ease into the day slowly, and stretch from sleepiness into readiness without rushing.

But from there, we dive in.

I know my student intimately—her energy, her patterns, her needs. On some days, Lucy can go full-speed through several subjects without missing a beat. On others, she needs a few extra breaks, a snack, a moment of quiet, or a walk around the block with the dogs. That's the gift of this kind of learning. It's not about being soft or avoiding hard things—it's about honoring the humanity of a child while still moving forward with intention. That same principle applies when Anderson is with us. His needs are different, but the heart behind our teaching remains the same: read the child, not the clock. Teach the student, not just the subject.

I believe that's one of the most powerful roles a parent can play—not just as a guide or facilitator, but as a steady, discerning presence. No one knows my children the way I do. And that intuition? That sacred, Spirit-led insight? That's part of the curriculum, too.

Of course, learning doesn't only happen at a desk. We've built our family values around experiences over excess, especially when it comes to birthdays. We call it "Places Instead of Presents." Sure, the kids still get a few thoughtful gifts—but the real gift is a trip, an adventure, a place to discover. We want them to walk the streets of new cities, taste new foods, hear unfamiliar languages, and marvel at the vastness of God's world with their own eyes. These aren't just vacations. They're immersive lessons in culture, gratitude, and awe.

It's one of the many ways we've chosen to flip the script—moving away from what the world says education should look like, and toward something deeper, more connected. Being both a mother and a teacher has shown me that knowledge sticks best when it's wrapped in a relationship. That discipline is most effective when it's rooted in love. That learning, at its best, is not about rushing through tasks but about forming souls.

Because in the end, homeschooling isn't just about academics. It's about discipleship. It's about teaching our kids to see truth, beauty, and goodness in the world—and in themselves.

And the light we raise in our homes? That's the light we leave behind.

Reflections Pages

1. A moment from this chapter that stood out to me:

2. How this moment connects to my own story, family, or childhood:

3. A belief, habit, or pattern I noticed in myself:

4. A more compassionate or truthful way of seeing this part of my story is:

____

____

____

____

5. One practical step I want to take this week is:

____

____

____

6. What might get in the way:

____

____

____

7. How I can support myself when it feels hard:

____

____

____

8. A Bible verse this chapter reminds me of and why:

____

____

____

9. A prayer, affirmation, or intention I want to carry forward:

____

____

____

Take what serves you, release what doesn't. Healing and learning are slow, holy work — and you are doing beautifully.

Part 5: Full Circle

As the dust of daily life settles, what remains? These final reflections look at the legacy of light we hope to leave behind—the kind that doesn't just shape childhood but ripples into generations. Because in the end, it was never just about raising children. It was always about raising hearts, raising faith, and raising light.

Chapter 22

For the Mama in the Aisle

"Therefore encourage one another and build each other up, just as in fact you are doing."

—1 Thessalonians 5:11

We've all seen her.

She's standing in the grocery aisle, trying to make a decision while her toddler wails. She's the one pushing a stroller with one hand, balancing a half-written list in the other, and praying that the goldfish crackers don't run out before she makes it to the checkout. She's in the school parking lot with tired eyes. She's at church, bouncing a baby on her hip and trying to follow the sermon with a preschooler clinging to her leg.

She's the mama holding it all together—and sometimes falling apart in the process.

If I could speak directly to her, I'd say this:

You're doing better than you think. I see the way you carry the weight of invisible things. The mental checklists. The guilt. The comparison. The fear that you're somehow not enough—or worse, too much. I see the love in your eyes, even when your patience is thin. I see the effort behind the exhaustion.

And I want you to know: you matter.

Not because of how clean your house is or how advanced your child is. Not because of what curriculum you chose or how many vegetables your kids eat. You matter because God handcrafted you to be their mama. And He doesn't make mistakes.

Your child doesn't need a perfect mom. They need a present one. One who keeps showing up. One who gets down on their level and looks them in the eye. One who apologizes when she's wrong. One who celebrates tiny victories and believes, fiercely, in who they're becoming.

And if you're in a season that feels lonely, misunderstood, or overwhelming—I want to remind you that you are not alone. This road you're walking is sacred ground. And the fact that you care so much, that you're even reading a book like this, tells me everything I need to know.

You're the kind of mama who's raising light.

So the next time you find yourself in that aisle—grocery store or otherwise—take a breath. You're doing holy work, even when it feels mundane. You're shaping souls, even when no one sees. And you are not walking alone. As this journey comes full circle,

I want to leave you with the story that ties it all together—the one that reminds me, every single day, why I choose to raise light.

Reflections Pages

1. A moment from this chapter that stood out to me:

2. How this moment connects to my own story, family, or childhood:

3. A belief, habit, or pattern I noticed in myself:

4. A more compassionate or truthful way of seeing this part of my story is:

____

____

____

____

5. One practical step I want to take this week is:

____

____

____

6. What might get in the way:

____

____

____

7. How I can support myself when it feels hard:

____

____

____

8. A Bible verse this chapter reminds me of and why:

9. A prayer, affirmation, or intention I want to carry forward:

Take what serves you, release what doesn't. Healing and learning are slow, holy work — and you are doing beautifully.

Chapter 23

The Light We Raise, The Light We Leave Behind

"Let your light shine before others, that they may see your good deeds and glorify your Father in heaven."

—Matthew 5:16

We don't get to keep them.

That may be the most bittersweet truth of parenthood. We raise them, shape them, pour ourselves into them—and then, little by little, we let them go. Into friendships. Into dreams. Into the world.

And if we've done it well, they won't need us the same way they once did. That ache? It's sacred. It means we did our job. Because we're not just raising children—we're raising future adults. Lights meant to shine far beyond the walls of our homes.

When I look at Lucy and Anderson, I often wonder: What will they carry with them? What phrases will linger in their hearts?

What habits will shape the way they love others? What truths will guide them when we're no longer nearby to whisper them?

I hope they carry not just the memory of love, but the way it was given. Freely. Fully. With laughter in the kitchen and forgiveness in the hard moments. With shared Scripture, unhurried walks, and prayers whispered over sleeping heads. I hope they remember that we didn't just talk about God—we relied on Him. That when things were beautiful, we thanked Him. And when they were broken, we still trusted Him.

I hope they remember that learning was more than academics—it was a way of life. That the greatest lessons weren't always found in books, but in moments: moments of character, of choice, of kindness. That we praised not just grades, but grit. Not just talent, but tenderness.

I hope they remember that we weren't perfect. Not even close. But we were present. We listened. We tried. And we never stopped believing that home was the training ground for the soul.

This journey of raising light—of watching it flicker, grow, and shine—has been the deepest honor of my life. But it didn't just transform my children. It transformed me. Motherhood became the classroom where I learned how to lead with grace, how to let go with love, and how to trade performance for purpose.

And now, as these pages draw to a close, I don't see it as an ending.

I see it as a beginning.

A full circle moment, where the child I once was—the one who struggled in school, who questioned her worth, who wondered if she'd ever find her place—has become a mother who creates that place for someone else.

If you're holding this book, I hope you feel a hand on your back, gently pressing you forward. I hope you feel seen, understood, and reminded that the work you're doing matters. Eternally.

Because one day, your child will walk into the world. And the light they carry will be shaped by the love, the truth, and the quiet faith you planted in them day by day.

We don't get to keep them.

But oh, what a legacy we leave behind.

Reflections Pages

1. A moment from this chapter that stood out to me:

2. How this moment connects to my own story, family, or childhood:

3. A belief, habit, or pattern I noticed in myself:

4. A more compassionate or truthful way of seeing this part of my story is:

____

____

____

____

5. One practical step I want to take this week is:

____

____

____

6. What might get in the way:

____

____

____

7. How I can support myself when it feels hard:

____

____

____

8. A Bible verse this chapter reminds me of and why:

____

____

____

9. A prayer, affirmation, or intention I want to carry forward:

____

____

____

Take what serves you, release what doesn't. Healing and learning are slow, holy work — and you are doing beautifully.

A Prayer for the Journey

Heavenly Father,

Thank You for the sacred gift of motherhood—for the honor of shaping lives, for the privilege of being a guiding light in the hearts of our children. Thank You for every ordinary moment that carries eternal weight—snuggles at dawn, books read aloud, scraped knees kissed, prayers whispered in the dark.

Help us, Lord, to parent with intention.

To trade performance for presence.

To see our children not as projects to perfect, but as souls to nurture.

Give us wisdom to lead, humility to learn, and courage to keep showing up, even when the days are long and the fruit is unseen. Help us to listen before we lecture, to pause before we react, and to love without condition.

May our homes be places where Your truth is spoken, Your joy is felt, and Your peace is known. May our children grow up knowing not just rules, but relationships—not just knowledge, but wisdom—not just love, but Your love.

When the world questions our path, steady us.

When we doubt our own ability, remind us that You are our strength.

And when we feel unseen in the quiet labor of parenting, remind us that You see it all.

Let the light we raise be a reflection of You.

And let the legacy we leave be one of faith, hope, and love.

In Jesus' name,

Amen.

Printed and bound in the United Kingdom
23/02/2026
02059163-0001